Planning Patient Care

FOUNDATIONS OF NURSING SERIES

WM. C. BROWN COMPANY PUBLISHERS

ANNA KUBA
Consulting Editor

Nursing Observation
Virginia B. Byers
Monroeville, Pennsylvania

Nursing Observations of the Young Patient
Margaret A. Coffin
Boston University School of Nursing

Promotion of Physical Comfort and Safety
Valentina G. Fischer and Arlene F. Connolly
Boston University School of Nursing

Promoting Psychological Comfort
Gloria M. Francis and Barbara Munjas
Medical College of Virginia

Problem-Solving in Nursing Practice
Mae M. Johnson, Mary Lou C. Davis, and Mary Jo Bilitch

Nurse-Patient Communication
Garland K. Lewis
Catholic University of America

Working with Others for Patient Care
Grace G. Peterson
DePaul University

Teaching Function of the Nursing Practitioner
Margaret L. Pohl
Hunter College

Planning Patient Care
Lucile Lewis
Loma Linda University

Planning Patient Care

Lucile Lewis
Loma Linda University

WM. C. BROWN COMPANY PUBLISHERS, *Dubuque, Iowa*

ISBN 0–697–05532–9

Library of Congress Catalog Card Number: 71-138563

Second Printing, 1972

Printed in the United States of America

PREFACE

This book is designed as a part of the Foundations of Nursing Series to serve as a textbook or reference for students of professional nursing. It is hoped that the book might also serve alone as a reference for the practicing nurse to assist her in planning patient care. Throughout the book, ideas are mentioned for nursing research and for the development of nursing theory or nursing science. The graduate student may profit from some of these suggestions.

Other units of the Foundations of Nursing Series explore in detail the observational capabilities of the nurse, the teaching function in patient care, the nurse's role in communication and in providing psychological comfort, and ways in which nurses work with others in providing health care. For this reason, some aspects of these essentials to the planning of patient care are not developed in detail in this book.

The basis for the planning of nursing care, whether for one patient or for a group, is the nursing process. An orderly, systematic way of looking at the person's needs for nursing provides the background for a nursing care plan which is patient-centered. The contents of this book are organized around the nursing process. My interest in the nursing process was awakened during my service on the Committee to Define Graduate Content in Medical-Surgical Nursing for the Western Council for Higher Education in Nursing. Work with that committee helped clarify my ideas about the nursing process.

The conceptual framework of nursing based on wholeness is still in a developmental stage. I realize that some of the elements of a theoretical framework are missing and must await additional thinking and clinical trial. However, because this concept seems to be particularly relevant to nursing, some aspects of the concept have been included throughout the book.

An effort has been made in this book to strike a balance between the ideal and the practical. However, some busy practitioners probably will disagree. No doubt, idealists will regard some of the practical suggestions as heresy. Because the planning of patient care takes time, the organizational pattern of hospital nursing may need adjusting to provide for this time. The trend in hospitals to transfer the clerical work done by team leaders and head nurses to ward managers and ward secretaries should give nurses the time they need to interview patients, to conduct planning conferences, and to study ways of improving patient care.

A large number of examples have not been prepared for this book. It is my belief that when a nurse knows the principles she can apply them in her own practice, adapting the principles to her own style of nursing. Those examples which are included are from medical-surgical nursing, because this is the area of nursing with which I am most knowledgeable.

The chapter on applying theory in practice is included because of concern for the gap which exists between theory and practice, between education and service. It is my belief that more effort should be expended by both education and service to narrow this gap and to put both education and practice on a firm scientific footing. Society has a right to expect this from professional nursing. The high cost of nursing services, as well as shortages in nursing personnel, might be offset by better planning and more effective use of nursing time. Better planning could increase the quality without increasing the quantity of nursing service, thereby facilitating a positive response in those who are served. In the end, this kind of care could lower the costs.

It would have been impossible to prepare this manuscript without sharing ideas and problems with my colleagues. The frank and constructive criticism of Mrs. Ina Longway is especially appreciated. For their suggestions, special thanks are due Ruth White, Beverly Steele, Aletha Fuller, Mary Pearce, and Pat Morris. A special "Thank you" also goes to Pat Clanton and her associates for their secretarial assistance in preparing the manuscript.

LUCILE LEWIS

CONTENTS

Chapter 1

The Nurse, the Patient, the Process

Planning of patient care is a complex process. It is complex because it may involve several people, perhaps of different disciplines, and it consists of several sequential steps built upon and logically derived from preceding steps. Adequate planning produces a set of actions designed to achieve one or more goals. The effectiveness of the plan must be evaluated in terms of the goals it was designed to accomplish. A plan for nursing care is more than a transcription to a special form of those acts of patient care delegated by the physician to the nurse. If nursing is a profession which offers services needed by humanity, then the plan should reflect the unique activities nursing can contribute to the welfare of people. The plan is a result of the combined efforts of nurses, patient, family, and other members of the health team to find ways in which nurses can assist the patient with his needs. Who is the nurse and what are the services that nursing can give? Who is the patient and what are his needs for nursing? By what process does the nurse work with the patient?

THE NURSE

The nurse who plans patient care is acting in her primary professional role—primary because the care of patients is the reason for the existence of nursing. Planning is professional since one characteristic of professional persons is their ability to identify and solve problems related to their field of practice.[1] The planning of patient care is actually a problem-solving process.

[1]Charlotte Towle, *The Learner in Education for the Profession,* (Chicago: The University of Chicago Press, 1954), pp. 3, 4.

The more educational and experiential preparation a nurse brings to the planning of patient care, the greater will be the scope of the problems she identifies, the more predictable and innovative will be the nursing actions she proposes, and the more objective will be the criteria by which she evaluates the nursing care she implements. If the preceding statement is true, the nurse responsible for the planning of patient care should be a person who has a college- or university-based education which has qualified her to practice nursing. Such an education should give her a background in the natural and behavioral sciences as well as in the humanities so that she has an understanding of the nature of human beings and appreciation and respect for the individuality of man. In settings where there are not enough fully prepared nurses, other nurses should be given the opportunity and guidance to develop planning skills to the full extent of their abilities.

Whatever her background, the nurse who plans patient care keeps her professional knowledge and expertise up-to-date by reading current publications; by attending inservice and continuing educational programs, regional workshops, and institutes; and by other available means of advancing herself. She brings to the planning of patient care an inquiring frame of mind, with which she is constantly seeking answers to the questions that arise. She has the courage to propose, carry out, and evaluate new approaches to patients' problems. The knowledge and expertise thus gained is shared with colleagues.

Service that the nurse renders to society is within the context of health and illness. Along with other professions, nursing aims to promote health and prevent disease. Health has been defined in a number of ways. Perhaps one of the best known definitions is that of the World Health Organization. "Health is a state of complete physical, mental, and social well-being, and not merely the absence of disease or infirmity."[2] Another concept of health is expressed by Hayman. "Health is optimal personal fitness for full, fruitful creative living."[3] If illness or disease represents anything less than the health implied by these definitions, and nursing operates within the context of health and illness, the scope of nursing is seen to be very broad.

In addition to the broad scope of health and illness problems, the nurse is prepared to work with patients in a variety of settings: in clinics or hospitals, extended-care facilities, private homes, and other places. While certain adaptations of care may be necessitated by the location of the patient, the essential nature of nursing care is common to all types of patient situations. Within the health/illness context there is room for the services of a growing number of professions. The nurse works with

[2]World Health Organization, Constitution of the, . Preamble.

[3]Howard S. Hayman, "Our Modern Concept of Health," *The Journal of School Health,* 32(1962):pp. 253-264.

persons from these other professions in meeting the health/illness needs of people and often performs tasks for patients which have been delegated to her by other health team members, but it is the caring functions of the nurse that are unique to the profession of nursing.

The Nature of Nursing

Caring implies that the nurse is concerned about what has happened to the health of the person and his family so that she wants to help them cope with their health and illness problems. Caring signifies those acts of ministration which help the person feel comfortable and safe. Caring helps the person retain his identity in a health/illness crisis. Caring means that the nurse is concerned about those things that concern the patient and she helps the patient find better solutions to these problems than he would have found alone. Caring is assisting the patient with those things he cannot do for himself or with which he needs help and doing them in a way that is acceptable to the patient. Caring is not only teaching the patient how to live with a disability but how to prevent further illness by living more healthfully. Caring is protecting the patient and his family from additional illness or injury. Caring is being concerned enough about the patient's responses to illness, hospitalization, therapy, and rehabilitation to help him maintain his integrity through such disruptions in his life patterns.

Caring is being observant for the clues that indicate a person is moving toward health or illness and initiating appropiate measures to enhance or retard these processes. Caring is maintaining a person's self-respect by helping him do all he can for himself. Caring is adapting nursing and other therapeutic measures to the patient's usual patterns of functioning whenever this does not jeopardize the outcome. Caring is being concerned for the continued progress of the person toward health when he is dismissed from the agency in which he contacted the nurse so that he leaves with a plan acceptable to him. Caring is supporting the strengths and alleviating the discomforts of the ill and the dying. Caring is discovering and providing the kind of environment which will facilitate the preventive and therapeutic efforts of all members of the health team for the restoration of the patient to his optimal level of health.

The caring nurse may insist on short-term discomforts to achieve worthwhile long-range goals. Caring provides anticipatory guidance to individuals and families for the prevention or early recognition of health/illness problems. Nursing is involved with families as well as individuals. The integrity of the family when it faces a crisis, the division of labor among family members when one member is incapacitated, the interaction among family members that promotes or retards the optimal development of each family member—these are examples of conditions about which the nurse cares and with which she helps the family cope.

Caring helps the underprivileged family cope with the problems of daily living. Caring means involvement with the safety of the individual and the family in the community. Nursing is concerned with keeping the environment free of pollution and contamination and with providing the kinds of health facilities needed by individuals and families. Caring helps individuals and families understand the importance of continued health supervision and how to obtain it.

Deviations in a person's health/illness status which necessitate his encounter with members of the health team are stressful to the individual. Engaging in diagnostic and therapeutic regimes may add to the stress of illness. Adjusting to a routine different from the patient's usual routine is upsetting, whether in the hospital, home, or extended-care facility. Caring finds ways to diminish the nature of these stresses and to alter the stress response. Caring is helping the person adjust to his situation and to cope with the adaptation. Caring is being concerned about maintaining the natural rhythms of the human being. These rhythms, timed by biological clocks, are chiefly synchronized by the daily routines of living. Altering these routines initiates a desynchronization of the circadian (24-hour) rhythms, adding more stress with which the person must cope. Caring means arranging the patient's daily program to keep it as close as possible to his usual pattern. Such an arrangement avoids adding the stress of desynchronized rhythms to the stress of illness.[4]

These caring functions are representative of the unique aspects of nursing. Nursing is concerned more with the effects of health or illness problems on the person or family and their reactions to the problems than with actual treatment of disease. Nursing is more concerned with the promotion of health and prevention of disease or disability than with cure.

In addition to the caring functions of nursing, the American Nurses' Association[5] has described two other components of professional practice as cure and coordination. Cure involves carrying out the therapeutic measures delegated by physicians and other members of the health team. The astute observations of the behavior of the patient, on the basis of which the therapeutic plan is maintained or changed, are part of the cure component of nursing. Helping the patient understand and accept all of the implications of his health problems in relation to his pattern of living is also a part of "cure."

Coordination is providing responsible leadership to all those who give nursing care. Nursing cannot meet all of the health/illness needs of people. The nurse, recognizing her limitations, is knowledgeable about community resources so that she can assist people to find the kinds of help they need.

---

[4]Gwen Jones Stephens, "The Time Factor," *American Journal of Nursing* 65:5 (1965):77-82.

[5]A. N. A. Committee on Education, "Education for Nursing," *American Journal of Nursing* 65:12 (1965): 106-111.

Coordination may involve arranging the services needed by a patient into a meaningful system.

Professional nursing practice is based on a conceptual framework which gives purpose and direction to practice, defines methods of practice, and determines relationships. Such a framework may be built upon the concept of wholeness. Many nurses endorse the concept of wholeness since the holistic response of man to life situations is confirmed by the nurse's association with people in varied life situations. In this monograph the concept of wholeness is seen as having two basic features. One feature of wholeness is its multidimensional unity in which all of the components interact in such a way that anything that affects one dimension affects all others. Some of the identifiable components of the whole are the physical, intellectual, emotional, spiritual, and social aspects of the total personality as well as the forces within the environment which impinge on the personality. In terms of the wholeness concept, a physical problem not only affects the physiological but also the intellectual, emotional, spiritual, and social components of the whole. Likewise, an impoverished social, spiritual, or emotional life affects all other dimensions. This aspect of wholeness conceptualizes the concern of nursing with the patient's multi-faceted reactions to health/illness problems.

The second feature of the concept of wholeness relates to the development of all of the individual's potentialities to the highest possible degree. It means he is working toward a more abundant life. Not too much is known about the potentialities that human beings can attain. Maslow has described a self-actualized man who lives at a high level.[6] Dunn in his treatise on high-level wellness defined individual, family, community, and social wellness and listed some criteria for evaluating wellness.[7] While these authors have made a real contribution to understanding of human potentiality, as new knowledge becomes available the nurse should seek to improve her understanding of this aspect of the concept of wholeness. In the present state of knowledge about human potentialities, perhaps the nurse can best apply this concept of wholeness by helping persons to understand the meaning of optimal total health and to formulate ways of working toward this state.

Nursing, then, endeavors to assist the person to accept wholeness as a goal and to plan a program of living consistent with the goal. Such planning will be influenced by a careful estimate of the optimal possible functioning of each dimension of the whole. The ability to estimate the potentiality of other persons improves with an understanding of the biological and behavioral characteristics of human beings, the environ-

---

[6]Abraham Maslow, *Toward a Psychology of Being* (New York: D. Van Nostrand Co., 1962), p. 24.

[7]Halbert L. Dunn, *High-level Wellness* (Washington, D.C.: Mt. Vernon Publishing Co., 1961,) pp. 159-200.

ment in which they function, and with careful evaluation of the nurse's past experience. The nurse orders her own life by the concept of wholeness so that she may serve as a model of health to those she serves.

The Roles of Nursing

In order to provide this kind of care, the nurse must function in a variety of roles as she works with persons needing her services. By helping a person in such activities as feeding, bathing, and exercising when he cannot perform them alone, she acts in a personal-service role. When the nurse explains to the patient or family how to prevent illness or how to adjust family meal patterns to include a therapeutic diet, she becomes a teacher in a teaching-learning situation. When she listens to a patient express his feelings about illness, disability, or other problems and helps him work out solutions, she acts as a counselor. In carrying out those functions delegated to her by members of other health professions, the nurse is usually performing in a technical role.[8]

Working with other members of the health team in planning, scheduling, and facilitating the patient's total program, the nurse serves as a coordinator, collaborator, and/or administrator. In the research role the nurse critically examines and analyzes all aspects of the nursing process and the reactions of patients to nursing care in order to contribute to the development of the nursing profession. When helping a person formulate and work toward goals of wholeness, the nurse employs her teaching and counseling roles. She continually searches for and tries ways of motivating people to accept and strive toward worthwhile goals.

Professional nursing has dependent and/or independent functions in relation to each nursing role. The dependent functions are those which are prescribed by the physician (or other member of the health team) and which are carried out by the nurse. The dependent functions of nursing form a large part of the "cure" component of nursing practice and the technical role. These include such functions as administration of drugs, assisting with treatments and diagnostic tests, collecting specimens for laboratory analysis, and the like.

Independent nursing functions are those initiated by the professional nurse. The "care" and "coordination" components, as well as some "cure" measures, are independent nursing functions. Examples of these are: the observation, recording, and reporting of effects of medications and treatments as well as the condition of the patient, teaching the patient how to prepare for a laboratory or radiological test and what he might expect as a result of the examination, arranging the patient's daily activities to coincide with his normal day as much as possible. Independent functions

---

[8]Hildegard Peplau, "Principles of Psychiatric Nursing," *American Handbook of Psychiatry*, Vol. II, Silvano Arieti (Ed.) (New York: Basic Books, 1959), pp. 1840-1856.

include helping a person adapt his therapeutic regimen to his usual pattern of living, planning and performing all aspects of personal hygiene the patient cannot do for himself, initiating protective measures to prevent the hazards of bed rest and the complications of disease or treatment. Control of the patient's environment, making referrals to other members of the health team and community agencies, teaching and counseling in relation to health and illness problems and preventable disease are all independent nursing functions.

In the process of evolving are new roles of nursing, among them the clinical specialist and the so-called "extended role." These new roles enlarge upon the independent functions of nursing. The clinical specialist confines her nursing activities to patients with problems in the area of her specialty. For these patients she assesses their needs, identifies their problems, and formulates short- and long-term goals. She systematically records her findings, goals, and prescribed nursing regime. Some particular aspects of nursing care requiring her knowledge and expertise are performed by the specialist; other aspects of care she may accomplish through organizing and directing the work of others. She evaluates the care she has prescribed and revises the program when necessary. She collaborates and consults with others in the care of the patient. The clinical specialist has at least a Master's Degree and can provide documentary evidence of her clinical competence and expertise in the area of her specialty.[9]

Areas of specialization are also in the process of evolving. Some seem to follow the medical specialty patterns—the cardiac nursing specialist, respiratory nursing specialist, and psychiatric nurse therapist. Others are based on age groups, such as pediatrics and geriatrics. Some specialize in such areas as crisis intervention, pain intervention, and nurse-midwifery.

The nurse clinician is a modification of the clinical specialist role for the nurse who lacks advanced academic preparation but who is a skilled practitioner in a limited field of nursing. Her skill has been acquired through guided practice and through continuing-education programs. At the present time, nurse clinicians are found in coronary and other intensive-care units and in psychiatric facilities.

The "extended role" of the nurse presently is identified with pediatric care. This nurse too has graduate preparation for her role which broadens and strengthens her abilities in observation and health evaluation. She can give compehensive care to the well child, can recognize developmental problems, and can manage some of the common problems of childhood. The pediatric nurse practitioner works in a variety of clinical facilities, independent of or in collaboration with a physician. It

[9]Committee to Consider the Position of Clinical Specialist, "Clinical Nurse Specialist Position Specifications," California Nurse's Association, mimeographed report No. 119, January 24, 1967.

is hoped that this extended role of the nurse will improve and expand the health care of chldren.[10] No doubt, as nurses are successful in this extended role with children, they may become involved in the health supervision of other population groups such as pre- and postnatal patients and ambulatory geriatric patients. In reality, these new roles represent refinement and strengthening of some of the traditional roles of nursing, perhaps with a narrow field of interest which is based on greater knowledge and skill.

As society continues to demand more and better health care, the roles of nursing will undoubtedly change to meet society's needs. Faced with these needs, it is the profession itself which must determine its direction and which must re-define nursing. Should the profession fail in this respect, so that other groups dictate what nursing is and is to become, the professional standing of nursing will be threatened. A profession worthy of the claim to professionalism must decide its own destiny.

THE PATIENT

The person who is the client of the nurse has traditionally been called the patient. The services of the nurse are needed by the patient because he has a health/illness problem with which nursing can help. The health/illness problem may or may not be obvious to the patient. He may be well aware of a problem which causes pain, discomfort, or deformity. He may not be aware that his diet is inadequate to maintain health, that his excessive smoking is dangerous to his well-being, or that his inability to give others responsibility is a factor in his teen-age son's delinquency. On the other hand, the services of a nurse may help a patient avoid a potential health/illness problem. Moreover, it may be necessary for the nurse to interpret nursing to the patient so that he is cognizant of the kinds of help he can expect from the nurse.

The patient who needs the services of nursing may be anywhere on the life continuum from conception to death. He may be at any point on the health/illness continuum from positive, abundant health to critical illness, hovering between life and death. The patient may be at any level of dependency, from total dependence on others to complete independence. Patients are human beings from all walks of life, the native and the foreign-born, the religious and the atheist, the affluent and the deprived. Patients are usually members of a family unit, and the nurse does not limit her services to the patient alone but considers the strengths and weaknesses of the family as a whole and how nursing can help the family work together for their common good. The nurse also is concerned about the forces in the community which affect the health of the patient.

---

[10]Susan Stearly *et al.*, "Pediatric Nurse Practitioner," *American Journal of Nursing* 67:10(1967):2083-2087.

Wholeness and Health/Illness Problems

When the patient is seen as a whole, the nurse is cognizant of the fact that what happens to one dimension affects the whole. The response of the person to a health/illness problem is unique to him in his life situation. The response is a response of the whole, not of a part. This means that the patient's medical diagnosis is not the only concern of the nurse. Her concern is with the total response of the person to the medical problem, its effect on his mental and spiritual health as well as on his family and other social relationships. Nursing is not alone in recognizing the need to minister to the "whole" man. In one of its brochures, the views of the American Medical Association are stated in this way: "It is widely recognized that a weakness in any of the four factors of health – physical, spiritual, mental or social – can and does militate toward illness in one or all three of the other factors. . . . Man is physical, spiritual, mental, social. He is a whole being, and in ill health, he requires total care and treatment."[11]

In terms of the concept of wholeness, a health/illness problem could arise when a person exhibits any lack of wholeness or imbalance among the various components of the whole. This lack or imbalance could arise from a difficulty or a perplexing situation involving any of the components of wholeness or from a breakdown in the interrelationships among the various components, such as a physical disease causing an unbalanced social response. The concept of wholeness also implies that the person is striving to reach his highest potential in all the components of wholeness and as a well-integrated human being. The person who is functioning at less than his potential can be said to have a health/illness problem.

Health problems are any difficulties experienced by the patient in maintaining and promoting his own or his family's health. Examples of such problem areas include: imbalance between food intake and the body's needs for nutrition, inadequate knowledge of the kinds of food necessary for good nutrition, a lack of knowledge of health services available, poor sanitation within the home, an unmet need for continuous medical supervision or a yearly physical checkup. Many health problems may arise from a person's or a family's lack of motivation to follow good health practices.

Illness problems arise when ill health of one or more components disrupts the whole. These problems include not only the disease process but also the signs, symptoms, and behavior changes occurring with the disruption of the whole. They involve the effects of illness on the person's total life situation, his family, his work, his social life, his religious life, and his reactions to these effects. Problems may also result from the

---

[11]Department of Medicine and Religion, *The Physician, The Clergy, and the Whole Man* (Chicago: American Medical Association).

person's reactions and responses to the illness or any aspects of his diagnosis, therapy, or rehabilitation or to his acceptance of the outcomes. Illness problems may occur within the patient's family because of the effects of the illness on the family's pattern of life, the change in role of the ill as well as that of other family members. Many problems follow the development of more or less permanent handicaps or disabilities caused by disease or trauma. Problems arise from all aspects of life and living that are directly or indirectly influenced by the status of the person's total health.

Health/illness problems may be present or potential. In other words the problem exists—there are data to support the fact of its presence. Other problems may not actually be present but data indicate a potential problem—the possibility that a problem might exist unless certain preventive measures are taken. It is important to recognize potential problems in order to carry out primary and secondary prevention. The potential problem of acquiring communicable diseases during childhood should lead to immunizations. The potential problem of pressure sores for the bedfast patient should lead to positioning, turning, and skin care procedures to prevent their development. Data about the patient which may provide clues to potential problems are as varied as the data on which identification of present problems is made. Common items to consider are the patient's age, educational and social background, former experience with illness, place on the dependency-independency continuum, the usual complications of his disease process, and his general health status. The epidemiological triad of agent, host, environment, and their interaction provide many clues to health/illness problems.

There are a number of variables which influence how an individual will respond to a health/illness problem. Culture defines health and illness in different ways and prescribes how the person deals with the problem. Culture determines the values important to a person and in other ways may delineate his potential development. Age, sex, and heredity may determine the diseases to which a person has a tendency as well as his level of health and response to disease. Socioeconomic conditions and environmental circumstances may not only be etiological factors in the development of health/illness problems but may influence the quality and quantity of health services available. Physical, intellectual, emotional, and spiritual development affect a person's response to disease and his capability of following a therapeutic or rehabilitation plan. The multiplicity and complexity of variables affecting the person (or family) are indicative of how well the nurse should know the patient if she is able to understand his responses and help him with his problems. All of these variables determine the potentialities possible to the individual in his present state of existence. The nurse continues to integrate into her nursing practice new knowledge pertaining to the effects of these variables on the health of the whole person.

The two-fold focus of nursing is (1) to help the patient and/or family cope with the physiological, intellectual, emotional, spiritual, and social reactions to health/illness problems and to maintain their integrity in the coping experience; and (2) to endeavor to move the patient (or family) toward a goal of optimal health of the whole personality.

There are many known ways of promoting health and preventing disease. When a person does not order his life in such a way as to be as healthy as his life situation permits, then the nurse helps him to understand how he can improve. She can point out the benefits of healthful living and in other ways attempt to motivate the person to work toward a higher level of health.

While the goal of optimal health may be seen by the nurse as a desirable objective, it may not be viewed in this way by the patient. The nurse and the patient may not agree on what the patient's potentialities are. They may overestimate these and then set unrealistic goals. The patient may have some ulterior motive for not living up to his capacities. In any event, the patient himself must be involved in appraising his own potentialities and setting his own goals.

The nurse helps the patient set goals by knowing the patient as an individual, by considering with him all that is known of the variables that set him apart as an individual. She helps him clarify his thinking, face reality, and consider the alternatives. The patient is free to accept, alter, or reject the goals, but the concern of nursing for the optimal health of the patient is a mandate to the nurse to present the patient with the knowledge that he needs to make an intelligent choice. It may be necessary to set initial goals at something less than the ideal. Success in reaching these goals may serve as incentive to set higher goals.

A deteriorating, irreversible condition of one component need not negate the possibility of wholeness as a goal. Wholeness for this person may be realized by building on his strengths to compensate for his weaknesses, by being mindful of the effect of the irreversible condition on his totality, and by supporting him in maintaining his integrity as a person.

It is recognized that it is inconsistent with the holistic concept to separate parts from whole. Yet it seems important to an understanding of the wholeness concept to specify the composition of the parts, the nature of health/illness problems, and the meaning of optimal health of the parts. These aspects of the parts are considered in terms of their application to nursing. Because of insufficient knowledge of the nature of man and his capacities, the whole is more than the sum of its parts. However, to understand the known parts should lead to some understanding of the whole.

Physical Component.

This component is the biological being. Since life is determined by the functioning of this part, it is basic to the whole. This part is composed of flesh and blood, organs and tissues—the anatomy and physiology. It is a growing, developing, changing organism from conception to death. Physical problems arise when a person is unable to perform the usual activities of daily living or when he does these in a way not conducive to health. Impairment of any body function creates a problem. Failure to grow and develop according to established normal patterns gives rise to physical problems. The prevention of impairments to which the person is susceptible is necessary to his physical well-being. The highest potential for physical health is not only absence of disease but a functioning of every system of the body at an optimal level so that the person has a harmonious sense of well-being. He has energy and vitality for an abundant life consistent with whatever physical limitations cannot be corrected.

Intellectual Component.

The ability to think and to learn comprises this component. Intellectual problems are created by disordered thought processes, underdeveloped or deteriorating mental ability, the need for stimulation, learning, and intellectual growth. Without intellectual stimulation, the mind does not reach its highest potential for wholeness, which is continued learning consistent with the mental abilities with which the person is endowed.

Emotional Component.

Emotions are a part of the totality of the individual. They are subjective feeling states which have both psychological and physiological components. Love, joy, fear, anger, grief are examples of emotions. With certain life situations, any emotion may be appropriate if its expression does not harm the person himself or other persons. Emotional problems arise when feelings expressed as a response to life situations are inappropriate to the situation or are harmful to the person or the groups within which he operates. Sometimes it is the behavior through which an emotion is expressed that is problematic, and the person needs to find more healthful ways of expressing his feelings. Optimal emotional health implies that emotions are appropriate to the life experience and are a true expression of the self. Healthful emotional expressions prompt behavior which is not harmful to the self or others. Perhaps this component, more than the others, determines the integrity of the whole by how constructively a person is able to cope with the vicissitudes of life, by how he faces reality, by his self-acceptance and his autonomy.

Spiritual Component.

The spiritual component of life revolves around a person's relationship to the object of his worship. To those who subscribe to the Judeo-Christian or Islamic faiths, God is the object of divine worship. Other beings, objects, or ideas are worshipped by people. Worship seems to be a common need of mankind—it is a need to relate to something greater than oneself. Who and how a person worships varies with the individual and the religion to which he subscribes. Whether or not the spiritual component of life fosters a more abundant life depends on the nature of one's God.

The highest quality of spiritual life is derived from a relationship with a loving, personal God Whose concern for the individual is that he will become all that it is possible for him to be. A loving, personal God is chosen by the individual as worthy of his trust and worship because He represents what is good and true in contrast to His counterpart's evil and error. A person's relationship to a loving, personal God gives meaning to life, a sense of belonging to the universe and eternity. This relationship enhances the individual's concern for the welfare of his fellow human beings. This kind of a spiritual life involves a personal commitment to God and an ultimate concern for a cause more lasting, more noble, and greater than oneself.

One's spiritual beliefs determine what he sees as right and wrong, the value he places on human life, the meaning of death, the nature of punishment for sin and reward for right doing. Health/illness problems have spiritual connotations because of these beliefs. When a person's life is inconsistent with his spiritual beliefs, guilt and other reactions can threaten his total health. Therapeutic programs may interfere with a person's usual pattern of worship and this may be a problem to him. The highest potential of spiritual health is a satisfying, growing relationship with a personal, loving God and a pattern of life consistent with one's beliefs. His beliefs are ever being examined in terms of truth.

Social Component.

The social dimension of life concerns one's relationship with other people, family, community, work groups, the world. Social behavior is determined by the norms of the society in which a person lives, the culture and ethnic groups to which he belongs. Social behavior is set by his status in society, his roles within his groups, and the social class to which his status ascribes him. The groups to which a person belongs define health and illness, prescribe appropriate activities, as well as set values on almost every aspect of life.

Social problems arise when a person's behavior is inconsistent with the behavior prescribed by his group, when he changes roles, when the values and norms of his group are inconsistent with those of the larger society. Problems may arise when a person's relationships with his groups are not satisfying, either to himself or to the group. Social problems produce stress reactions which involve all the components of the whole. Physical and/or mental illness impose social problems when a person must change roles, accept new roles (such as patient, dependent, amputee), or alter his value system. Social problems may be an etiological factor in a number of illnesses. John Donne, the poet, displayed great insight when he wrote, "No man is an island." The highest potential of social health is satisfying group relationships in a social order which permits growth of the individual as a person and which values his contribution to the community.

The Environment.

The person is influenced not only by the physical aspects of his environment (temperature, humidity, microorganisms) but by the social forces within the community (economic, political, technological). Social forces determine the kind and extent of health care available to the person; the safety and degree of contamination of the food, water, and air he needs; the kind of housing available; the protection from harm (war, crime, injury). Both physical and social aspects of the environment are etiological factors in many diseases. Environmental forces may enhance or deter the therapy and rehabilitation of diseases.

Environmental problems exist when physical and social conditions in the environment cause ill health or deprive the individual or groups of the basic human rights of life, health, liberty, and happiness. A healthy environment is one which is safe from climatic, chemical, and microbiological hazards, from war, crime, poverty, and accident. It is a community in which the individual is free to develop to his highest potential commensurate with the constraints imposed upon him by his own limitations and for the common good of society.

THE PROCESS

The process by which the nurse identifies, plans, and implements the nursing care of the patient is a problem-solving process which can be defined in three steps: assessment, intervention, and evaluation.

Assessment is a complex phase in which data concerning the patient are collected and sorted into appropriate problem areas. These problems are examined in relation to the nurse's philosophy of nursing and policies of the agency in which she practices. They are then stated as problems with which the nurse can help. Priorities among problems are determined.

Intervention consists of both planning and giving care. With the patient's problems in mind, nursing objectives are formulated as statements of desired outcomes in patient behavior as a result of nursing care. A number of actions may be proposed for each objective, and from these the nurse must select those actions which seem most suitable for the individual patient. If those alternatives selected do not achieve the objectives as planned, then others will be initiated.

Evaluation is the phase of the nursing process by which the nurse uses measurable criteria to learn whether the nursing objectives were accomplished. If the actions did fulfill the objectives, those actions are included in the nursing-care plan. If the actions selected were not appropriate to the objectives, then they will not be retained in the nursing care plan and the patient will be reappraised and other actions derived.

The nursing process will be examined in more detail in subsequent chapters.

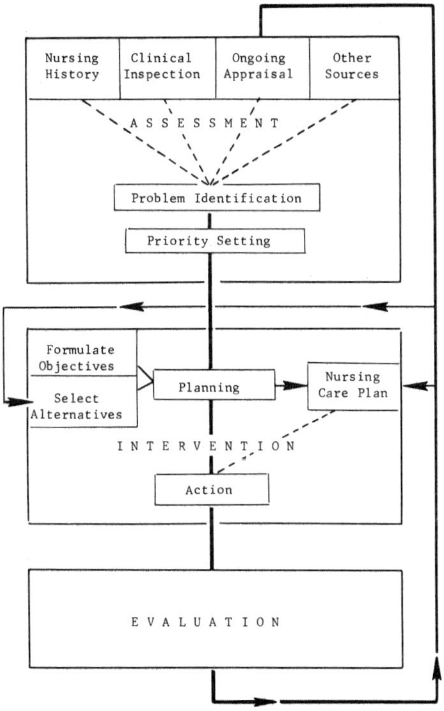

Figure 1.1. The Nursing Process

REFERENCES

*A.N.A. Committee on Education. "Education for Nursing." *American Journal of Nursing* 65:12(1965):106-11.

*Dunn, Halbert L. *High-Level Wellness.* Washington, D. C.: Mt. Vernon Publishing Co., 1961.

Engel, George L. "A Unified Concept of Health and Disease." *Perspectives in Biology and Medicine* 3:4(1960):459-85.

Glover, B. H. "A New Nurse Therapist." *American Journal of Nursing* 67:5 (1967): 1003-5.

*Hayman, Howard S. "Our Modern Concept of Health." *Journal of School Health* 32(1962):253-64.

*Suggested for additional reading.

*Johnson, Dorothy E. *et al.* "The Clinical Specialist as a Practitioner." *American Journal of Nursing* 67:11(1967):2298-2303.

*Levine, Myra E. "The Pursuit of Wholeness." *American Journal of Nursing* 69:1(1969):93-8.

*Lewis, Lucile. "This I Believe about the Nursing Process–Key to Care." *Nursing Outlook* 16:5(1968):26-9.

*Little, Dolores. "The Nurse Specialist." *American Journal of Nursing* 67:3 (1967):552-6.

Maslow, Abraham. *Toward a Psychology of Being.* New York: D. Van Nostrand Co., Inc., 1962.

*Murray, Louise B. and Barnard, Kathryn E. "The Nursing Specialist in Mental Retardation." *Nursing Clinics of North America* 1:4(1966):631-40.

Mussallem, Helen K. "The Changing Role of the Nurse." *American Journal of Nursing* 69:3(1969):514-7.

Neilson, Norma J. "The Clinical Specialist in a Rehabilitation Center." *Nursing Clinics of North America* 1:3(1966):365-73.

Otto, Herbert A. "Research in Human Potentialities: Implications for Public Health Nursing," mimeographed paper, University of Utah.

*Peplau, Hildegard. "Principles of Psychiatric Nursing." *American Handbook of Psychiatry* (Vol. II, Silvano Arieti, ed.), New York: Basic Books, Chap. 92(1959):1840-56.

Provonsha, Jack. "Wholeness–an Idea Whose Time Has Come," mimeographed paper, Loma Linda University.

Schlotfeldt, Rozella. "A Mandate for Nurses and Physicians." *American Journal of Nursing* 65:12(1965):102-5.

*Smith, Dorothy M. "Myth and Method in Nursing Practice." *American Journal of Nursing* 64:2(1964):68-72.

*Sobel, David E. "Human Caring." *American Journal of Nursing* 69:12(1969): 2612-3.

*Stephens, Gwen Jones. "The Time Factor." *American Journal of Nursing* 65:5(1965):77-82.

Stokes, Joseph, III, *et al.* "Physicians' Assistants." *American Journal of Nursing* 67:7(1967):1441-4.

Tillich, Paul. "The Meaning of Health." *Perspectives in Biology and Medicine* 5(1961):92-100.

Vaughan, Margaret D. "The Role of the Clinical Specialist in Surgical Nursing." *Nursing Clinics of North America* 3:3(1968):507-14.

CLINICAL EXPERIENCE

1. Observe practicing nurses functioning in a variety of roles. Record activities which pertain to each role.
2. Observe nurse-patient interactions and describe caring functions.
3. Interview patients to find out how their illness has interfered with their life situation.
4. Interview patients regarding their usual health practices.
5. Observe a clinical nurse specialist and a staff nurse in a similar clinical setting. Compare their activities and roles.

---

*Suggested for additional reading.

Chapter 2

Tools and Skills of Nursing

Essential to each occupation are some characteristic tools and/or skills which enable the practitioner to perform the functions of his trade or profession. The carpenter has his hammer, plane, and level. The farmer uses tractors, plows. The seamstress, needles and thread, patterns, and sewing machine. The surgeon, scalpel, hemostats, dissecting scissors. Some of the tools of various occupations are in the form of hardware. Other tools and skills are in the realm of interpersonal relationships, decision-making, and group leadership. Like other professions, nursing has some tools and skills which are vital to the practice of nursing.

When the nurse is planning patient care, she must consider the tools and skills that both she and her team members have available to them. Not only does the nurse use some inanimate tools in the practice of nursing, she also uses herself as a person and some management skills in the planning and giving of patient care.

INANIMATE TOOLS

In addition to the hardware nurses use in all steps of the nursing process, certain printed forms and other paper goods have a real place in the practice of nursing.

Equipment and Supplies

Equipment and supplies used by the nurse vary with the different agencies in which the nurse works. Examples run the gamut of the contents of the public health nurse's bag, the school nurse's bandaids, posters, and audiovisual teaching aids, the hospital nurse's dressings, thermometer, sphygmomanometer, respirators, and disposable supplies.

Some equipment may be used in the assessment phase to gather information, in the intervention step as therapy, or in the evaluation of care to denote change. A tape measure may be used to determine the circumference of an edematous extremity as a part of assessment, and it may be used to evaluate positioning to relieve edema. A stethoscope may be used to assess the condition of the patient's lungs; it may be used to evaluate the effectiveness of deep breathing and coughing or tracheal suctioning. A urethral catheter may be used to find whether a patient has residual urine; it may be used as intervention for retention of urine. Equipment and supplies used in nursing intervention include disposable syringes and needles and dressings as well as respirators, hypothermia machines, prosthetic devices.

Equipment is as simple as a tape measure or a thermometer or as complex as an Engstrom respirator or a computer. New devices become available with such rapidity that it is difficult to keep abreast of developments. One reason for the need for continuing education is the rapid development of new supplies and equipment. It is essential that the nurse know how to operate and to make the best use of all the equipment used in the particular branch of nursing in which she practices.

Important as supplies and equipment are, they are only tools which the nurse uses to accomplish a purpose. The nurse must be ever mindful of this and must not become so fascinated with the machinery that the interpersonal relationship between nurse and patient becomes meaningless.

The Nursing Care Plan

Another tool useful in carrying on the practice of nursing and coordinating nursing efforts into a meaningful whole is the nursing care plan.[1] The nursing care plan serves as a guide for giving nursing care. It is a compilation of the nursing objectives which are formulated for the patient and of the nursing actions to be carried out. It lists those functions delegated to nursing by the physician or other health team members.

The nursing care plan is a written form which contains all current information regarding the nursing care of the patient. The form may be a 5 x 8-inch file card placed in a *Kardex* file. Some cards are 9½ x 8 inches folded to 5 x 8 inches to make more surface available. Other forms may be filed in a loose-leaf notebook or other device for keeping the nursing care plans of a group of patients together and the plan for an individual patient separate.

The printed form used for nursing care plans is divided into several sections. Most forms include: (1) an area for general care – the physical

[1]The content of the nursing care plan is discussed in Chapter 5.

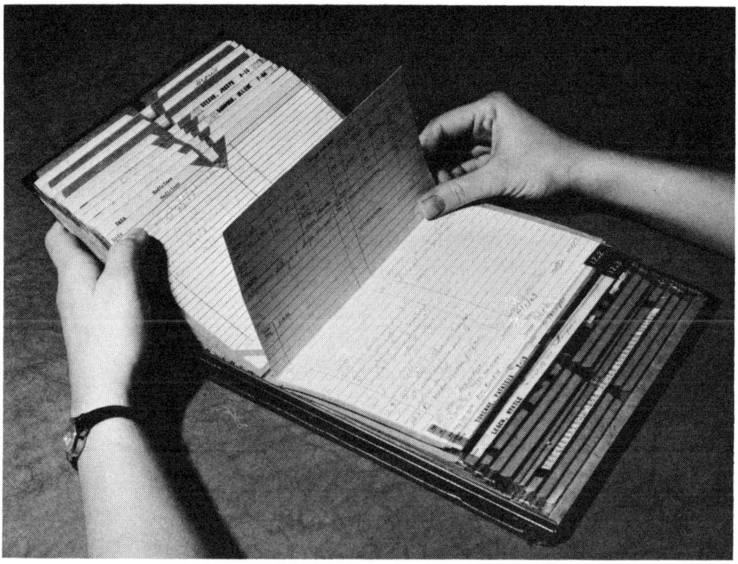

Figure 2.1. A Kardex File for Nursing Care Plans
Note the surfaces available for recording items of nursing care.
Card 1 is an 8" x 5" card placed on the back of the preceding card.
Card 3 is an 8" x 9½" card fitted into the file space. It is folded to 8" x 5" size, with a fold-over flap, Card 2.
Card 2 is the flap of Card 3. Both sides can be used.

and safety needs of the person and personal hygiene measures, (2) an area for medications and treatments prescribed by the physician, (3) a place for patient's appointments, and (4) a section for nursing objectives and independent nursing actions. Provision is also made for listing the statistics of the patient – such as name, age, religion, diagnosis, room number, physician. The format of nursing care plans should be adapted to the requirements of the agency in which it is used. Some way should be devised to assure that nothing is overlooked when writing the care plan, and there should be room on the format to develop those parts of the care plan which are most pertinent to a particular patient.

It is the responsibility of the team leader to formulate the original plan of care, to keep it up-to-date, and to include those items necessary for the discharge plan. The planning that goes into the preparation and up-dating of the care plan is shared by the team leader and the nursing team.

Properly used, a nursing care plan is a tool which can assure continuity of care for the patient. All nurses concerned with the care of the patient refer to it as a guide for the giving of patient care. Examples of formats for nursing care plans are shown in Figures 2.2 and 5.2 (pages 20 and 100).

MEDICAL-SURGICAL NURSING CARE PLAN I ICH 880

PERSONAL HYGIENE
____ Spec. Mouth Care
____ Comp. Bed Bath
____ Bed Bath c̄ Help
____ Tub Bath
____ Shower

BOWEL-BLADDER
____ Bedpan-Urinal
____ BRP c̄ Help
____ BRP
____ Commode/BM
____ Catheter
____ Incontinent

EATING
____ In Chair
____ Feeds Self
____ Assist
____ Feed

DEXTERITY
____ R or L Handed
____ Impaired

ACTIVITY
____ Comp. Bed Rest
____ Bed Rest c̄ BRP
____ Dangle
____ Up in Chair
____ Amb. c̄ Help
____ Amb. ad lib

PREVENTIVE CARE
____ Bed Board
____ Bed Cradle
____ Foot Board
____ Trapeze
____ Turn q ____ hrs.

PROSTHESIS
____ Glasses
____ Contact Lenses
____ Dentures:
Upper ____
Lower ____
Partial ____
____ Hearing Aid

BEHAVIOR
____ Confused
____ Wanderer
____ Withdrawn
____ Noisy

INTERESTS
____ Hand Crafts
____ T.V.
____ Radio
____ Games
____ Books

SPEECH
____ Aphasic
____ Foreign

HEARING
____ Impaired
____ Deaf

VISION
____ Impaired
____ Blind

Write date if Dr.'s order
✓ if nursing diagnosis

NAME

MEDICAL-SURGICAL NURSING CARE PLAN II ICH 881

Adm. Date: Time: AM/PM	Age: Birthday:	Religion	Marital St. M S D W	Spec. Reports & Date Sent

Dx. Adm.: Sec.:	SURG. Date: (In Red)

ASSESSMENT OF PATIENT NEEDS	NURSING APPROACH	PATIENT INSTRUCTIONAL NEEDS

Acuity Category 1 2 3 Condition: Last Rites:

Name	Dr.	Hosp. No.	Room

Figure 2.2. Nursing Care Plan: Inter-Community Hospital—Medical-Surgical Wards, 275 West College Street, Covina, California 91722. Used by permission.

The Patient's Record

The patient's record serves not only as a source of information for the nurse in assessing the patient's needs but as an account of the nursing care he received. Notations made by the physician may provide clues that the patient's nursing needs should be reappraised. The physician's notes may also contain evidence to use in evaluating nursing care. Besides the physician's notes, the data from the clinical laboratory, X-ray Depart-

Date	GENERAL NURSING CARE	Interval
	Weight	
	Blood Pressure	
	Temp-Pulse-Resp.	
	Neuro Check	
	Intake/Output	
	Diabetic Urine	
	Foley Cath.	
	Isolation	
	Other	
	Daily Lab. Work	

Date	DIET & FLUIDS
	Food Allergies **(In Red)**
	Extra Nourishment ☐ None Allowed ☐ Diet Kitchen ☐ Floor Kitchen

Date	TREATMENTS	Interval

ALLERGIES — Other than Food or Drug **(In Red)**

MEDICATIONS

Date Order	Date Exp.	PAIN RELIEF	Interval	Date Order	Date Exp.	SCHEDULED MEDICATIONS	Interval
		SLEEP					
		OTHER P.R.N.					

DRUG ALLERGIES **(In Red)**

Name	Dr.	Hosp. No.	Room

Figure 2.2. (Continued)

ment, consultations, and other services, can give valuable information for the assessment of the patient's needs and the evaluation of nursing care.

Entries in the nursing section of the patient's record should include assessment data, what the nursing actions were, and an evaluation of the action. The nursing history should be a part of the patient's permanent record. Since nursing care plans are temporary, changing guides to nursing care, and not usually a part of the patient's permanent record, the nursing notes on the record should give evidence of the contents of the nursing care plan. The problems identified, the nursing objectives, and approaches to those objectives should be a part of the permanent record. Changes in approaches as well as the reasons for the changes should be included. This kind of information is invaluable in planning future care of the patient. It gives the nurse a firm basis for selecting alternative courses of action in the solution of current problems. She can learn from the record what has been tried before and how well it worked. With these data as guidelines, she should be able to make more reliable predictions of the outcomes of the actions she recommends.

Entries in the patient's record should provide dependable data for nursing research. The usefulness of patient's records for research will be assured only if entries contain descriptive assessment data, accurate accounts of nursing action, and objective evidence that the nursing actions were evaluated. Nursing notes should be so accurately kept that they will provide clear evidence if submitted for legal action.

The nursing audit committee is usually commissioned with the responsibility of checking that physician's prescriptions for nursing care were carried out and that the routine care of the patient was accurately and completely recorded. One activity of the nursing audit committee might be to verify from the nurse's notes that the nursing care plan was indeed carried out.

Computers

The computer is becoming an important tool in many health agencies, although nursing has scarcely begun to make use of this space-age wonder. It is being used in some agencies for preparing staffing schedules. Storage and retrieval systems are being used for storing information about patients and making selected information available on request. To transcribe physician's orders for medications, laboratory or X-ray procedures, diets and other services, a few keys may be punched by the nurse at the nurse's station. Immediately a print-out is available for the nurse to check whether the correct message was put into the machine. Upon punching another key, the information is stored in the computer and the respective departments concerned with the physician's order receive print-outs. Computers compile medication lists for the nursing unit for each hour that medications are given. Instead of recording on the patient's chart that she gave the drug, the nurse punches a key and the computer records the fact. An alarm system is activated if the computer does not receive the information that the drug was given. Much other paper work, such as census reports, lists of critically ill patients, lists of available beds, can be taken over by the computer. Programming a computer to do much of the routine paper work should free nurses for direct patient care.

Some people envision the computer as an aid in improving nursing care and job satisfaction of nurses by matching patient needs with quality and quantity of nursing personnel.

From well-developed nursing care plans, the total nursing activities for a group of patients could be fed into a computer. In turn, the computer could indicate the number and types of nurses needed for the specific group of patients. Staffing could, in this way, be adjusted to the actual needs of the service. Likewise, print-outs could itemize the nursing actions required for each patient for a given time period. Many of the notations that nurses must customarily write on the patient's record could be key punched and the print-outs could be added to the record. Electronic monitoring and continuous recording of the vital signs is another capability of the computer. Many nurses have discovered the capabilities of the computer as an aid to nursing research.

No doubt, imaginative nurses will continue to find ways that the computer can serve them by extending themselves, by performing routine tasks, by supplying selected information needed for decision-making, or by manipulating data for the solution of problems. Relieved of such tasks, the nurse should develop her assessment, planning, and interpersonal skills to capitalize on the human aspects of nursing care.

THE NURSE HERSELF AS A TOOL

Nursing is interpersonal in nature – it is a helping relationship in which the nurse helps the patient in various ways. While the nurse sometimes uses tangible tools in the helping process, she often uses herself. To speak of the nurse as a tool tends to depersonalize her, but this implication is by no means intended. Indeed, it is the warmth of the nurse's own personality, her manifest interest in the patient, that make her a therapeutic person.

The Nurse's Hands

In all three steps of the nursing process, the nurse uses her hands. With her hands, she can feel skin texture, detect temperature changes, and operate devices for obtaining physiological data about the patient. With her hands, the nurse helps the patient with various aspects of personal hygiene. Her hands give support and assistance with moving in bed, position change, and walking. The nurse's hands apply various bandages, packs or dressings, massage body parts, give medications in any of several methods. Manual skills are required to operate suction, breathing, resuscitation, and irrigation equipment. And with her hands, the nurse may obtain objective data for evaluation of nursing care.

Through the medium of touch, the nurse may use her hands to communicate comfort, safety, and supportive messages to the patient. The manner in which a nurse uses her hands, either in the operation of equipment or in touching and helping the patient, may be therapeutic. The smoothness with which she does things, the degree of skill manifested, the gentleness and firmness of her touch contribute to trust and comfort. The way a nurse uses her hands may say to the patient "I care," "I know what I'm doing and why," "I believe this will help you,"– or something short of these messages.

The Nurse's Senses

Her own senses are the tools the nurse uses for observation. With her eyes she notes color, texture, form, movement, position, spatial relationships, expression. Hearing includes not only the spoken words, but enunciation, tone of voice, and choice of words. Her ears also pick up sounds emitted by the body, such as heart and breath sounds and peristaltic activity. Her sense of touch reveals to the nurse temperature, texture, moisture, vibrations, size and shape, tension. Odors of various body secretions and excretions as well as environmental conditions stimulate the sense of smell. While a sense of taste is important to the nurse herself, its relevance to nursing is minimal.

Observation of the patient on a continuous or periodic basis has long been considered an important function of nursing. It is quite possible that physicians regard this as the most important function of nursing. Be that as it may, observation of the patient's behavior is both a dependent and an independent function. Often the physician prescribes the particular aspects of patient behavior he wants the nurse to observe and record. In addition, it is an independent function of the nurse to use her knowledge and skill to observe and report the significant aspects of the patient's physiological and psychosocial behavior. The nurse should be competent to decide how often these behaviors need assessing and what she should do with the information. This kind of observation may more accurately be called perception, since perception implies an understanding of what is perceived by the senses.

Types of behavior which the nurse observes are varied and cross all the components of wholeness. She observes physiological behavior by noting pulse or respiratory rate and rhythm as well as many other signs and measures. Psychosocial behavior is marked by attitudes, moods, and interactions with people. Vocal and bodily expressions may indicate emotional, spiritual, or social problems. Symptoms may be a manifestation of deviant physiological or psychosocial functioning.

The perceptive nurse is ever sensitive to expected as well as unexpected developments with the patient. Her observations are not so mechanical or stereotyped as to blind her to the unforeseen or unpredicted. She always maintains an attitude of conscious awareness, sensitivity to change. The significance of any change in behavior is suspect until proved otherwise.

Intelligent observation of the patient is essential for the collection of data for planning. It is an essential aspect of the care implemented, and it is crucial to the evaluation of care.

The Nurse's Health

As suggesed in Chapter 1, the nurse may act as a model of health for the patient. Her health practices and her own healthy personality can serve as an example to the patient. It is incongruent to think of an obese nurse helping a patient to understand that obesity is a high-risk factor in heart disease or diabetes. Neither does it seem consistent for a nurse who is a chain smoker to discuss the possibilities of chronic obstructive lung disease or lung cancer with a chain smoker. Nor is an anxious nurse, full of bitterness and hostility, apt to help another person cope successfully with anxiety. To sell positive, abundant health to a patient or family, the nurse herself should be as healthy as it is possible for her to be.

The Nurse's Personality

Because of its interpersonal nature, the nurse's own personality is an influential feature of the nurse-patient relationship. The nurse is not all things to all people, but as a nurse her primary function of caring fosters healing. The nurse is not some model of excellence set apart from other people, but she does care enough about people to become involved with them. The caring functions of nursing[2] can only be performed by a person who is concerned for the welfare of others, who has insight into the meaning of life's experiences for the other person as well as for herself. The loneliness of illness can be made bearable to a patient by a nurse who understands what he is experiencing, whose interest in him as a person conveys strength and confidence. The stark realities of poverty may be brightened by a nurse who can show the way to help, who respects the person so much that his own self-respect is enhanced. The appeal of health in a healthy, happy nurse can motivate others to incorporate into their own lives those behaviors which promote health.

Empathy, openness, out-goingness are almost trite expressions in nursing literature. Yet their relevance to nursing, to the helping relationship between nurse and patient, assume more and more importance as nursing attempts to define its unique role in patient care. These are the characteristics of the nurse which promote a healing, trusting nurse-patient relationship.

To perform the caring functions of nursing, the nurse must be free to be herself, to not be so molded by professionalism that her own unique

[2]See Chapter 1.

personality is distorted. The nurse must have self-respect and self-confidence and must care enough about herself to gain the respect and confidence of her colleagues as well as of her patients. In the practice of her profession the nurse should seek and her employer should provide an environment conducive to the continued growth and development of her personality.

MANAGEMENT TOOLS

Essential to the person who is responsible for the planning and implementing of patient care are some management tools. These tools help people work together toward common goals. They may be used to effect change. These tools can help people grow so that each person's contribution to the service is enhanced and his personal satisfaction with his work is heightened. Communication is both an art and a skill. It is a way through which the nurse uses herself as a therapeutic person. Communication is also an important part of working with others. For this reason, communication is presented here as a bridge between the nurse's use of herself as a tool and the tools of management. Other management tools contributing to planning patient care are team nursing and leadership.

Communication

Communication refers to the process by which thoughts, ideas, attitudes, and feelings are transmitted from one person to another. Communication may be verbal, an exchange of words, or nonverbal, where ideas are conveyed by gestures, touch, facial expression, distance, posture. Communication occurs "whenever there is a meeting of meaning between two or more persons."[3] The derivation of the words communication and communion is similar. Therefore, communication implies involvement, fellowship, an intimate relationship of mutual trust. Only with this kind of communication can there be a meeting of meaning.

There are four elements of communication. These are (1) a sender, the person who originates the communication process; (2) the message, the idea, thought, or feeling that is conveyed; (3) the receiver, the person who accepts the message; and (4) feedback, the way in which the sender determines whether the receiver got the message he intended. Communication has not occurred unless all of these elements are included in the process. In a given communication, one person alternates between sender and receiver. Feedback is the one element missing from many attempts at communication, and without it the effort is merely an attempt. A short circuit exists in the communication cycle and the cycle is incomplete when there is no feedback.

[3]Reuel L. Howe, *The Miracle of Dialogue* (New York, Seabury Press, 1963), pp. 22-23.

Without feedback it is impossible to know what message the person received, since both verbal and nonverbal language may not be interpreted in the same way by the sender and the receiver. Feedback is just as important in nonverbal as in verbal communication. Often, the sender assumes that his message got through to the receiver but does not find out for certain whether it did. Such assumptions often lead to misunderstandings, to actions based on improperly interpreted directions, or to conclusions not based on facts. For the nurse to understand her patient, for the leader to understand her followers or to be understood by them, the communication cycle must be unbroken. Like the message, feedback can be either verbal or nonverbal.

The art of listening is vital to the process of communication. To listen effectively, the receiver must give his entire attention to the sender. Attentive listening is manifest by facial expression and eye contact as well as by verbal responses. The listener must discipline himself to concentrate on what is being conveyed by the speaker and must not let his mind wander to other things. His interest in what the other person is communicating must be genuine. Pretended interest, no matter how subtle the pretense, is always obvious to the sender, and communication is blocked. The listener's whole being must be focused on the other person.

Active listening searches for both the literal and the intended or implied meaning of what is said. The receiver is aware of consistencies or inconsistencies between the spoken word and the tone of voice, facial expression, mood, or other form of nonverbal expression. When the listener notes inconsistencies, he seeks clarification so that he actually receives the intended message. Occasionally, the listener may summarize

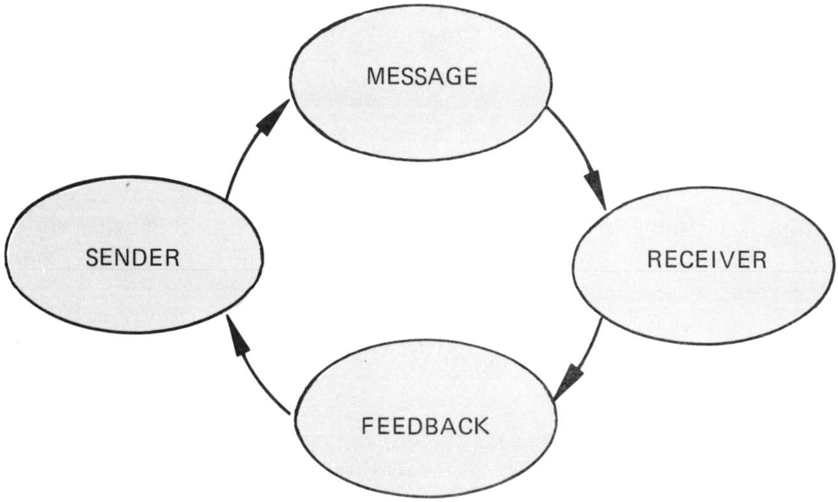

Figure 2.3. The Communication Cycle

the message he has received so that the sender can verify it. At other times when it is necessary to verify or clarify the message, the receiver may reflect key words or phrases, paraphrase them, ask an open-ended question, or indicate in some other way that the message is not clear. Techniques such as these give the sender feedback and let him know the response of the receiver to what he is saying.

It has been said that, since we have two ears and only one tongue, we should listen twice as much as we talk. This admonition applies both in the nurse-patient relationship and in the leader-colleague relationship. One can learn a great deal by listening, whereas when he talks he is merely expressing what he already knows.

Involved listening makes the speaker feel important, it raises his self-esteem. In turn, the speaker's regard for the listener is enhanced; he feels that here is a person who can be trusted. The nurse who is a good listener can readily develop rapport with her patients as well as with her co-workers. Listening is one way for the nurse to show that she cares.

The nurse's awareness of her own and of the other person's personality increases her perception of the thoughts, feelings, attitudes, and behavior of both sender and receiver and thereby enhances communication. Likewise, the nurse must be cognizant of the barriers to communication so that they can be removed, controlled, or dealt with in some other way. Howe defines a barrier to communication as "something that keeps meaning from meeting."[4] Barriers to communication are set up by language, culture, and age differences. Anxiety, dissimilar aims and purposes, and the defense mechanisms a person uses may also act as barriers.

Unless manual skills are accompanied by communication, the patient becomes an object to which things are done rather than a person who needs the help of the nurse. Communication with the patient may be used without manual skills, but manual skills should rarely be used as a nursing action without concurrent communication. Except in lifesaving emergencies and in a few other unusual situations, each act which the nurse performs for a patient should be preceded by an explanation of its purposes and its effects on the patient. The nurse should provide opportunity for feedback, for the patient to ask questions about what she is doing and to offer suggestions which might make the nursing action more acceptable to him.

Communication skills are indispensable to both the nurse-patient relationship and to the management roles of the nurse.

Team Nursing

One system of providing for the nursing needs of people is an organizational tool – team nursing. Basic to this concept is the utilization of

---

[4]Howe, *The Miracle of Dialogue,* p. 23.

different levels of nursing personnel to meet the needs of a group of patients. Nursing tasks are distributed among the team members in accord with their abilities and preparation. Nursing personnel range in ability and preparation from the on-the-job trained nursing assistant through the licensed vocational or practical nurse, the registered nurse with a diploma, associate or baccalaureate degree, to the nurse with clinical specialization on a graduate level. Because of differences in education, experience, native ability, personality, and commitment to nursing as as profession, there are no sharp and distinct lines between the various levels of nursing. Some nurses function far above that for which their education has prepared them, others considerably below. Many nurses have a high potential for growth with continuing education, and they may learn to function adequately at a level above their basic preparation. The shortage of health service personnel compels all administrative nurses to encourage each nurse to develop to her highest professional potential.

Figure 2.4 illustrates the types of nursing tools and skills commonly performed by the various levels of nursing personnel. The diagram shows that those with the least preparation use mostly simple, inanimate tools; their management skills and ability to use themselves therapeutically are less well developed. Those with the most preparation use fewer, more complex inanimate tools, perhaps of limited variety. They are more skilled in the therapeutic use of the self and in management. In between, where most nurses fall, is possible a wide range of skills, some more, some less developed. Some of these nurses are good leaders, many are excellent followers. There can be no leaders without followers. Followers are the nurses who are the backbone of the profession; they are the caring people most involved in actual patient care.

Inherent in the concept of team nursing is the group approach to planning and to nursing action. The group works together, each member of the team contributing her part to the nursing care of the patients. Team conferences and ward rounds are essential components of team nursing. Both may be used to plan or to evaluate nursing care. Both may be used to improve nursing care by discussing those qualities and techniques needed to improve performance. These group activities may be helpful in coordinating the efforts of the nursing and health teams.

The team conference is a meeting of the members of the nursing team for the purpose of planning and organizing the day's work, discussing and designing the nursing care of a patient, or acquainting all members with some new problem or procedure. The team leader usually leads out in the team conference. The patient may or may not be present.

Ward rounds, conducted by the team leader, consist of visits to patients by all or part of the nursing team. These contacts aid in the planning of patient care by involving the patient and the nurses in some aspect of

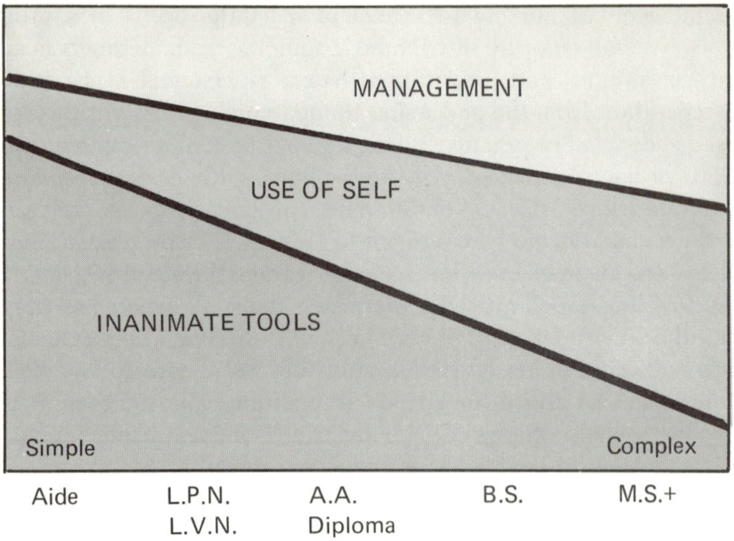

Figure 2.4. Types of Nursing Tools and Skills Used by Different Levels of Nursing Personnel

the planning. The team leader may wish to assess the patient's condition with those who will be giving direct care to the patient so that all have a common understanding of what to observe, what the baselines are. She may use this occasion to plan which team member is responsible for different aspects of care. She may demonstrate how to carry out some therapeutic measure and may discuss with the team members how to evaluate the measure and what to enter on the patient's record. The nurses may explore with the patient how he wants his care done and what he thinks will help him most. Never should nursing rounds be conducted "over" a patient, treating him as an object rather than a person. The main purpose of ward rounds is to involve the patient in his care, to help him express his needs and the manner in which he would like these met. Having ward rounds is one way of communicating the patient's needs to all nurses giving him care.

Another way of facilitating the team approach to patient care is for the team leader to accompany the physicians on medical rounds. Visiting patients with medical staff gives the nurse an opportunity to learn more about the physician's plan of therapy, the progress of the patient, and what the physician tells the patient. Knowing what the physician tells the patient gives the nurse a background for helping the patient truly understand what the physician said to him. Also she can encourage the patient at this time to discuss with the physician those things he needs to know. By participating in the doctor-patient relationship, the nurse can better coordinate the patient's care in order to attain the goals set for him. An understanding of the patient's total regime is essential for the planning of patient care.

The team approach to patient care can be strengthened by the use of consultants and specialists. Whenever they are available, knowledgeable people should be consulted in order to help nurses understand and interpret data about the patient. The intelligent use of resource persons can elevate the practice of nursing in a way similar to continuing educational programs. Consultants and specialists can contribute to experiential learning by nursing personnel. These people can help nurses identify patient problems and develop innovative and purposeful solutions to those problems.

Leadership

Leadership is the ability to guide and direct the work of others, initiate action, to mobilize for the achievement of a purpose. A degree of excellence and competence as a practitioner is expected of a leader. Of necessity a leader must have followers; in nursing these followers are the members of the nursing team. Teamwork is working together as a group to achieve a goal. Teamwork can only succeed with effective leadership, willing and cooperative followers, and goals accepted by the group as worthy of their efforts. To effectively plan and implement nursing care, a nurse needs certain leadership skills.

Planning is a function of leadership. Planning is working out in broad outline the things that need to be done and the methods for doing them to obtain the desired objectives of the service. Effective planning achieves objectives at minimal cost and effort. It analyzes all the elements involved in meeting goals. Planning simplifies jobs so that all unnecessary factors are eliminated.

The leader is acquainted with the strengths and weaknesses of each of her workers and she assigns them tasks for which they are best suited. The leader is interested in the professional growth and development of her workers and she uses every opportunity to foster their growth. She is interested in them as individuals, in the satisfactions they derive from their work, in their personal aspirations or problems which influence their work. She is concerned about both the quality and the quantity of her staff, and she works with them and with her supervisors in planning patient care so that the staff is adequate to meet the objectives of patient care.

An essential skill of the nurse-leader is coordination of the work of the team so that similar complementary activities are arranged in logical groups, and overlapping and duplication of functions are avoided. This kind of coordination facilitates a smooth-running unit. It is one way of accomplishing the most with the least. Coordination involves inter-relating the parts to the whole, synchronizing the various components of the effort in relation to time, place, and persons so that each will fit into the total program. "Coordination is the orderly arrangement of group effort, to provide unity of action in the pursuit of a common purpose."[5]

Another leadership skill needed by the nurse is the ability to give orders. To do this, she not only needs effective communication skills but she must be able to direct the work of others, to get others to do what she asks them. This must be done in a tactful, democratic manner, using requests rather than demands, and being explicit in stating the request. The feedback element of communication is vital when giving orders. Feedback enables the leader to know that the person to whom she gave the order understands it. Since the leader has the authority to give certain kinds of orders, she must also assume responsibility for seeing that the order is carried out. She must follow through and know that the task has been completed.

Leadership in nursing requires teaching capabilities. The team leader teaches her team members how to perform certain aspects of nursing care. She adapts teaching methods to the learner, the content, and the situation. Her own professional competence and excellence are utilized in teaching others to improve their nursing abilities. The nurse also teaches patients, individually and in groups. She helps patients change their ways of living if change is needed to improve health. She assists them in adapting to a therapeutic or rehabilitation program. Teaching includes the setting of goals for learning and the evaluating of the change in behavior resulting from the learning process as well as communicating information necessary to achieve the goals.

The leader is aware of her place in the organizational structure within which she works. She is able to work in a collaborative relationship with those in line positions as well as in staff positions to accomplish the goals of nursing. She keeps those to whom she is responsible informed about what is going on. As a nurse, she is also responsible to her profession. She keeps herself and her colleagues aware of professional issues. She shares her knowledge and experience in any way she can to advance the profession of nursing. She interprets nursing to the community.

The nurse team-leader is aware of the costs of operating the agency in which she works. She plans and coordinates her part of the program to the advantage of the total effort. She contributes to this effort by the proper care and maintenance of equipment, the economical use of time and supplies, avoiding waste and duplication of effort. Her interest in developing her workers to their highest potential, in minimizing tardiness and absenteeism, and in the efficient use of time serve to benefit the organization.

---

[5]Wm. R. Spriegel, "Coordination . . . The Key to Management Teamwork," *American Association of Industrial Nurses' Journal,* 4(1956):26-31.

In a nursing situation, the leader accepts the philosophy of the organization and uses it as a guide for her nursing functions. She is also aware of her own philosophy of nursing as an influence on her practice of nursing and of leadership.

Leadership is an essential tool for the nurse who plans patient care.

* * * *

The craftsman is proud of his tools and keeps them in good working order. He keeps them sharpened and polished. He obtains new ones as they are developed. He uses each one for a designated purpose. The nurse may learn a lesson from the care a craftsman gives his tools and should do all it is possible for her to do to keep the tools of nursing sharpened and polished and up-to-date. Day by day, she can improve her skill in using these tools, ever learning from her practice. In this way, her competence will be improved and the satisfaction she derives from the practice of her profession will be enhanced.

REFERENCES

*ALMAN, BEATRICE. "Patients Participate in Nursing Care Conferences." *American Journal of Nursing* 67:11(1967):2331-4.

BAIN BARBARA. "The Therapeutic Role of the Staff Nurse." *Nursing Forum,* II:2(1963):90-7.

CHRISTMAN, LUTHER B. "Nursing Leadership—Style and Substance." *American Journal of Nursing* 67:10(1967):2091-3.

DEMARCO, JAMES P. "Automating Nursing's Paper Work." *American Journal of Nursing* 65:9(1965):74-7.

EDELSTEIN, RUTH R. "Automation: Its Effects on the Nurse." *American Journal of Nursing* 66:10(1966):2194-8.

*FLYNN, EILEEN D. "The Computer: An Aid to Nursing Communication." *Nursing Clinics of North America* 4:3(1969):541-8.

*HOWE, REUEL L. *The Miracle of Dialogue.* New York: Seabury Press, (1963): pp. 3-35, 51-66.

*JOURARD, SIDNEY, M. *The Transparent Self.* New York: D. Van Nostrand Co., Inc., Part V(1964):111-55.

*KRON, THORA. *Nursing Team Leadership.* Philadelphia: W. B. Saunders Co., 1966.

*LEWIS, GARLAND K. *Nurse-Patient Communication.* Dubuque, Iowa: Wm. C. Brown Company Publishers, 1969.

MCKINLEY, JEAN E. "Inservice Education for Leadership." *Nursing Outlook,* 16:9(1968):47-9.

*MELODY, MARY, and CLARK, GENEVIEVE. "Walking-Planning Rounds." *American Journal of Nursing* 67:4(1967):771-3.

MERCADANTE, LUCILLE T. "Leadership Development Seminars." *Nursing Outlook* 13:9(1965):59-61.

NORTHRUP, LINDA. "Conferences Mean Better Nursing." *American Journal of Nursing* 66:6(1966):1342-3.

PARRAMORE, BEATRICE, and YEAGER, WAYNE. "Team Nursing in Public Health." *Nursing Outlook* 16:6(1968):54-6.

*Suggested for additional reading.

*PETERSON, GRACE. *Working with Others for Patient Care.* Dubuque, Iowa: Wm. C. Brown Company Publishers, 1969.

*PRICE, ELMINA. "Data Processing—Present and Potential." *American Journal of Nursing* 67:12(1967):2558-64.

RAMPHAL, MARJORIE M. "This I Believe About Excellence in Technical Nursing." *Nursing Outlook* 16:3(1968):36-8.

RAUFFENBART, MARY. "Drug Administration by Automation." *Nursing Clinics of North America* 1:4(1966):611-20.

ROWAN, ROBERT L. "Automation: Its Effect on the Hospital." *American Journal of Nursing* 66:10(1966):2199.

*SISTER REGINA ELIZABETH. "The Team Assignment Plan." *Hospital Progress* 46:2(1965):76-82.

*SPEED, EUNICE L. and YOUNG, NANCY A. "Scan—Data Processed Printouts of a Patient's Basic Care Needs." *American Journal of Nursing* 69:1(1969): 108-10.

SWANSBURG, RUSSELL C. "An Experiment in Team Nursing."
Part I, *Nursing Outlook* 16:8(August, 1968):45-7.
Part II, *Nursing Outlook* 16:9(1968):42-3.

TARRANT, BETTY JANE. "Automation: Its Effect on the Patient." *American Journal of Nursing* 66:10(1966):2190-4.

WALKER, VIRGINIA H. and HAWKINS, JAMES L. "Management: A Factor in Clinical Nursing." *Nursing Outlook* 13:2(1965):57-58.

WEIL, THOMAS P. and WEIL, JANET W. "The Use of Computer Systems in Patient Care." *Nursing Forum.* V1:2(1967):207-17.

WOOD, M. MARION, *et al.* "The Team Conference." *Nursing World* 134:3 (1960):9-10.

CLINICAL EXPERIENCES

1. Observe the practicing nurse to determine which tools she uses to meet the various needs of patients.
2. Listen to a nurse-patient or nurse-nurse conversation to identify the four components of communication. Identify the missing components when the communication was ineffective.
3. Find out how computers aid nursing in one clinical facility.
4. Observe the nursing roles performed by various levels of practicing nurses on one team. Indicate the tools most used at each level.
5. Consider a recent nurse-patient situation in which you were involved. Which tools did you use for different purposes. Were they appropriate? Why?
6. Observe or conduct a team conference and/or ward rounds and evaluate the effectiveness of the session in terms of planning patient care.

*Suggested for additional reading.

Chapter 3

Assessment—Data Collection

Planning of patient care is dependent upon a body of information about the patient, his family, and his environment. This information points out needs of the patient for nursing care and serves as a basis for planning. Planning follows a careful assessment of the patient. Assessment is the first step of the nursing process, yet it also may be carried out simultaneously with the other steps of the process. New data about the patient may be obtained during any interaction with him. While assessment is a more or less continuous phase of the nursing process, it must always precede intervention and evaluation. The second and third steps cannot be performed in a meaningful, personalized manner unless based on data pertinent to the patient. Actions performed on the patient without a proper assessment are mechanical, stereotyped actions which are not designed to meet the needs of the individual. Such actions may or may not be harmful.

Assessment consists of the collection of data about the patient and the identification of his nursing problems or needs. Assessment is a complex perceptual and interpretative function. It is based on broad knowledge, astute observation, and purposeful listening. It is essential to the initiation of the plan of care for the patient. The quality of the plan of care can only be as good as the assessment on which it was based.

Data for assessing the needs of the patient are obtained from several sources. These sources will be examined separately. The nursing history comprises data concerning the patient's patterns of functioning at the initial meeting of the nurse and her patient. The clinical inspection yields data pertaining to the physical condition of the patient when he is first seen by the nurse. The on-going appraisal is continual collection of data relevant to the changing needs of the patient. Other sources of information vital to formulating a nursing care plan are the patient's medical record and the literature upon which the nurse's knowledge is based. All these data must be sorted and categorized in order to identify the nursing problems of the patient. Once the problems or needs are identified, they are ranked in order of priority.

THE NURSING HISTORY

Purpose of the history is to obtain information needed to personalize nursing care of the patient. The nursing history establishes the patient as an individual who has likes and dislikes, fears and hopes, reactions and expectations, habitual patterns of functioning with which he is comfortable, and some degree of competency in the various components of wholeness. The information in a nursing history is essential to the caring functions of nursing. This history may also point out areas in which the patient is or is not approaching his highest potential for wholeness. With this information the nurse may plan teaching and counseling designed to help the person achieve a higher level of wholeness. Data from the nursing history may partially or fully support the existence of nursing problems.

At the initial encounter with the patient, the nurse interviews him for the purpose of obtaining information for the nursing history. Ideally, the nurse who obtains the nursing history should be the team leader responsible for his nursing care. If the patient's condition is critical, if the patient is a child or is in some way incompetent to give a lucid history, the nurse obtains the information from a family member. Even though most of the information can be given by the patient, an interview with the family often provides meaningful information. The response of the family members to the nurse's questions, as well as the interaction of the patient and family, give the nurse important clues as to the effect of the patient's illness on the family. Other clues may indicate the kind of support the family can give the patient, the family resources available to help the patient, and the needs for help which exist among family members.

Content

What kinds of information should be included in the nursing history? Primarily, it must be information particularly pertinent to the nursing care of the patient, not a repetition of a medical or social history. Time, personnel, and finances are too limited to waste patient and nursing time in unnecessary duplication of effort. The content of the nursing history will reflect the philosophy of the nursing service of the agency as well as the nurse's own beliefs about the nature of nursing. If the nurse sees herself as primarily dependent on the physician for direction of care, her nursing history will be considerably different from that taken by a nurse who sees herself as a caring person concerned with the patient's reactions to his health/illness experience, as a person who adjusts the patient's new routines to his familiar patterns, and who initiates measures which promote health and prevent complications.

Information recorded in the nursing history must be of the type that nurses can use in the planning and giving of nursing care. For instance, there is no need to know the time of day a patient prefers some aspect of his care unless the timing of his care is flexible and can be adjusted to his wishes. If the agency prescribes that all baths be completed before 11:00 a.m., there is little need to know whether a patient prefers an evening or a morning bath. If no adjustments can be made in the way meals are served, there is no need to find out what times the patient prefers to eat or which meal he prefers to have as his largest or smallest meal.

Some information from the medical and social histories is important in planning nursing care. The nurse must judge within the context of her own situation whether it is more advantageous to her and/or the patient to obtain this information from the patient or from the record. Usually, the information borrowed from the medical or social history will have to be expanded in such a way as to make it relevant to nursing. For instance, there may be a notation in the medical history that the patient complains of insomnia. Knowing this, the nurse may say, "The doctor noted on your chart that you have trouble sleeping. Tell me more about this . . ." The fact that the patient has insomnia is not enough information to plan nursing care. The nursing history should include answers to some of these questions: At what hour does the patient usually retire? arise? What does he do to prepare for bed? What activities make him sleepy: music? reading? hot drink? warm bath? Does he have trouble getting to sleep or does he awaken in the night and then have difficulty getting back to sleep? How much sleep does he get during the day? The answers to these questions are not found in a medical history, yet they would be invaluable in planning care to meet the patient's need.

The word *history* implies something that has preceded the present. It is past. The nursing history contains information about the patient's past experience and usual habits which may influence his nursing care. This information is not something that changes as his health status improves or deteriorates. The information in the on-going appraisal will reflect the changes in his condition. The nursing history may include comments regarding the patient's anticipations of the consequences of his health/illness experience. These expectations are brought by the patient to the nurse-patient encounter and may color his behavior during the remainder of his experience with nurses and other health personnel.

General content of the nursing history reflects (1) the reactions and expectations of the patient regarding his health/illness situation, (2) his usual patterns of functioning, and (3) his competencies in each of the components of wholeness. Reactions of the patient to his present and past health problems, to his hospitalizations, diagnostic tests, and therapeutic programs take the form of emotions and attitudes as well as signs and symptoms. The expectations of the patient influence his behavior as well as determine his acceptance or rejection of the therapeutic plan. How the patient responded in the past and responds in the present to his health/illness experience give clues to his methods of coping with stress, his needs for information, his willingness to follow a therapeutic regimen, his attitude toward health service personnel.

In order to make as few changes as possible in the patient's habits of living, an inquiry is made into the patient's usual patterns of functioning. Pattern of functioning is defined as the characteristic or usual ways in which a person performs the activities of life – the things he does in his usual day, the order in which he does them. These patterns of functioning concern food and fluid intake, elimination, rest and sleep, exercise, personal hygiene measures, and responses to pain and discomfort, as well as other patterned responses to daily living. One listing of patterns of functioning is given in the Summary of Assessment Data, pages 57-62.

Competence[1] refers to the patient's capacities to meet his own needs in the various dimensions of wholeness. Competency levels are estimates of the strengths and weaknesses of the whole person and/or each component of wholeness. Competencies are derived from knowledge of the patient obtained in the nursing history interview and from the clinical inspection as well as from other sources of information. Physical competence refers to the general status of the patient's physical health, his dependence on others, on drugs or other measures, or on prostheses for the maintenance of his health. Physical competence should also consider the person's ability to carry out prescribed therapeutic, rehabilitative, or preventive measures. Mental competence pertains to the person's ability to understand, to relate cause and effect, to solve problems, to recall near and distance events. His educational and language background affect his mental competence. Emotional competence is evidenced by emotional maturity, the ability to make and carry out decisions, to assume responsibility for one's own behavior. Spiritual competence is concerned with the strength of one's religious faith, by his dependence on faith and religion in everyday life and in crises. Social competence refers to family integrity, the respect, support, and love given other family members, the

[1]This term is adapted from that used in the "Family Coping Index" developed by Johns Hopkins Hospital School of Public Health and the Richmond (Virginia) Visiting Nurse Association.

Ruth B. Freeman and Marie Lowe, "A Method for Appraising Family Public Health Nursing Needs," *American Journal of Public Health* 53:1(1963):47-52.

sharing of family responsibility. Social competence also depends on the quality of performance of work, social, and family roles. Environmental competence relates to the availability of needed health services; the safety, space, and privacy provisions in the home; transportation facilities; and chemical and bacteriological safety.

While interviewing the patient and family for the nursing history, the nurse uses this opportunity to assess their mental and emotional status. The nurse asks herself: Are remarks consistent, appropriate, and relevant to the questions asked? Is language facility consistent with age and educational background? Is affect appropriate to the occasion and to the topics discussed. Are nonverbal expressions suitable? Do mannerisms show undue nervousness or anxiety? Are there some topics they seem hesitant to discuss or some which are overemphasized?

The preceding discussion on nursing history is somewhat idealistic in approach. It may be adapted to a given situation by focusing on high priority areas of need, by establishing a policy regarding types of patients who will have complete nursing history, those who will have high priority areas explored, and those who may have no history at all. For instance, in hospitals, the patients who are admitted ambulatory for a diagnostic work-up may not need a complete nursing history. This does not imply they have no nursing needs or that their needs are unimportant. For practical reasons, these patients are probably better able to manage with less nursing care than are other patients. Two truths should be considered by the nurse before she consigns thorough nursing histories to the realm of the impossible. "Where there is no vision, the people perish."[2] "A nurse cannot practice beyond the boundaries of her own vision."[3]

There are times when the acuteness of the patient's problem precludes obtaining a satisfactory nursing history. In such instances, the nurse may have to base her actions on clinical inspection alone and/or obtain only that information particularly applicable to the presenting problem. If and when the acuteness of the condition lessens, additional information can be obtained so that a more complete plan of care can be devised.

It is economical of time, effort, and thought to classify information for the nursing history in the same way that the nursing care plan is arranged. When writing the nursing history, all of the data regarding rest and sleep should be in the same part. Likewise, all of the data about exercise, food and fluid intake, elimination, or any other item should be gathered together. This way of organizing the data facilitates identification of problems and transcription of information to the nursing care plan.

In addition to the sample nursing history forms (pages 41, 43-45, 47-49), the Summary of Assessment Data (pages 57-62) gives examples of

[2]The Holy Bible, Proverbs 29:18, King James Version.

[3]Katherine J. Bordicks, *Patterns of Shock* (New York: The Macmillan Company, 1965), p. 21.

question topics that a nurse might use for a nursing history. These questions are presented as topics only, since the nurse will want to phrase the questions in a way suitable to her, to the patient, and to the situation. The list is not considered all inclusive. Nor is it meant to imply that any one patient would be asked all of these questions. It is quite possible that, for any one patient, only a small number of areas of inquiry will need to be explored at length. Each nurse will want to ask questions in a manner which is consistent with her own personality and philosophy of nursing, and she can adapt her questions to the language ability, intellect, and physical condition of the patient.

Methods

There are at least three approaches which the nurse might use to obtain a nursing history. Which type is chosen depends on the time available, the policy of the agency in which the nurse and patient meet, and the preference and capability of the nurse herself.

Probably the least desirable form would be a questionnaire which the nurse asks the patient to fill in. The chief advantage of this method is its time-saving function for the nurse. If time is not available for a more thorough type of nursing history, then this method is preferable to having no history at all. Its chief disadvantage lies in the fact that the nurse gets few clues to problems which conversation with the patient might reveal. The questionnaire does not permit adequate exploration of the facts about the patient nor about his feelings. Neither does this method contribute much to the development of trust and rapport between patient and nurse. A questionnaire tends to be routine and stereotyped, not personalized to the patient. (Fig. 3.1, p. 41.)

A second method of obtaining a nursing history is an interview schedule. This may list actual questions which the nurse will ask the patient and it provides space for the answers or it may merely list topics for questions which the nurse will phrase in her own way. This method of obtaining the nursing history allows for more individuality than the questionnaire, and it provides some opportunity for further exploration of areas in which problems are seen to exist. A form for this type of nursing history was developed by McPhetridge.[4] The interview schedule gives structure to the nursing history and gives some assurance that information on desired topics will be secured. It may serve as a helpful guide for the new nurse or the student of nursing until she develops her own style for obtaining the nursing history. Whether the nurse's writing down of the patient's answers to questions in his presence blocks communication is debatable. Perhaps no straightforward decision can be made since the personalities of both patient and nurse influence their reaction to this

[4]Mae McPhetridge, "Nursing History: One Means to Personalize Care," *American Journal of Nursing* 68:1(1968):68-75.

NURSING HISTORY

Questionnaire

To Patient or Family Member: Mrs. G. L.
Please complete this questionnaire so that we may adapt your nursing care to your wishes. Thank you.

Is this your first hospitalization? no, 3rd If you have been in hospitals before, what did you like about the care? interested nurses

What did you NOT like about the care? being fed by tube

What do you expect as a result of this hospitalization? able to eat again

Who will help you when you leave the hospital? husband

Do you ever have trouble getting your breath? no If so, what brings this on? ____ What do you do when this occurs? ____

Does your heart ever pound or skip beats? no If so, what brings this on? ____ What do you do when this occurs? ____

What time of day do you have your meals? usually 7³⁰, 1, 6-7 Snacks? no

What do you usually eat for

Breakfast? Noon Meal? Evening Meal? Snacks

Have been on sustagen tube feedings for 2½ months. 1 cup 6 times a day

What foods or drinks do you not wish to be served? soft drinks

What foods or drinks do you especially like? all - when I can eat

Estimate the number of glasses (cups) of fluid you drink each day 6-8

Do you have any problems urinating? no Do you have to get up at night to urinate? occasionally How many times? once

How often do your bowels move? once a day What time of day? around 9 am.

Do you ever have constipation? no Diarrhea? no

What do you do to treat constipation or diarrhea? ____

What is your usual time of going to bed? 11 pm Arising? 7 am

Do you sleep well? usually If not, what do you do to help you sleep? ____

What do you do to get ready for bed? wash up. listen to news on radio

How many pillows do you use? one - soft How many blankets? 2 - 1 electric

How much exercise do you get every day? walking around house

Are you right handed? X left handed? ____

Do you ever have pain? no Where is the pain? ____

What do you do to relieve the pain? ____

What kind of bath do you prefer? (Tub?) Shower? Time of day to bathe? morning

When do you prefer to brush your teeth? after breakfast, bedtime

Do you have dentures? no When do you wear them? ____

What brand of dentifrice do you prefer? Crest Mouthwash? Listerine

Do you have any trouble speaking? no Seeing? no Hearing? a little

Describe Hear better with left ear

Do you wear glasses? yes Contact lenses? ____ Hearing aid? ____

What do you do for recreation? read, knit, write letters Hobbies? my dog

What would you like to do for diversion while ill? read, listen to radio

What church do you attend? none

If you wish your clergyman to visit you, what is his name? Chaplain OK.

Are there any people you would especially like to visit you? husband

Are there any you do NOT wish to visit you? no

If there are any other wishes concerning your care, please explain below

Can't sleep in strange places. Like it quiet.
Like back rub at bedtime.
Skin very dry. Apply Lubriderm lotion after bath.

Figure 3.1. Nursing History Form

or any other type of interview. In the interest of saving time, a combination of the questionnaire and the interview schedule or semistructured interview may prove efficacious in a given situation. (Fig. 3.2, p. 43.)

It would seem that the most desirable method of taking a nursing history is the semistructured interview. In this instance the nurse has in her mind a general outline of all the kinds of information desired for the history. She uses open-ended questions to obtain data from the patient. Being alert to clues to nursing problems, she is free to explore these in detail with the patient until she is satisfied with the data obtained. Actual practice often discloses that only two or three areas of inquiry need exploring in depth with any one patient. During the interview, the nurse may write a few brief notes to support her memory. After the interview she records the nursing history. The chief drawback to the semistructured interview is that it may require a fairly large segment of nursing time. The flexibility of the semistructured interview is one of its prime advantages. It can be adapted to the patient and to the nurse to allow for free expression of feelings, attitudes, and beliefs in relation to the facts of the patient's life experiences. The feelings, attitudes, and beliefs which the patient expresses during this type of interview indicate his values and provide more clues to the type of person he is than do the mere facts of his life. Armed with these clues, the nurse should be able to personalize his nursing care more appropriately. Furthermore, the interest shown in the patient by the nurse in providing time for him to express himself freely should go a long way toward developing understanding of the patient as a person and creating mutual trust and rapport between patient and nurse. In considering the feasibility of using this method of obtaining a nursing history, the initial time requirement should not be the only criterion. It is possible that taking time at the introductory nurse-patient encounter for a thorough history may eventually save time as well as contribute to the satisfactions and health of the patient. A thorough nursing history should enable the nurse to identify more nursing problems, to make a significantly better nursing care plan, and to implement nursing measures which make better use of nursing time, enhance the patient's rehabilitation, and may even shorten his period of care. (Fig. 3.3, pp. 47-49.)

In any one agency several types of nursing history may be used. The format might be determined by the stage of illness of the patient, his dependency state, the nature of his needs for care and education, the acuteness or chronicity of his need for care. Whatever method is used the nurse should remember that the history-taking interview is an information-gathering interview, not a counseling session. The qualifications of the nurse in the different areas of the agency would also determine the type of history used. A clinical nursing specialist should be expected to take

NURSING HISTORY

Interview Schedule

REACTIONS AND EXPECTATIONS Mr L. C.

What is the reason for your hospitalization? heart attack

What do you expect from this hospitalization? to get well

What effect has your illness had on your family? spoiled plans to go to Hawaii

Have you had previous hospital experiences? yes

Was there anything you especially liked about the care? no

Anything you disliked? bland diet

What are your feelings about examinations and treatments? OK. if necessary

PATTERNS OF FUNCTIONING

Do you ever have difficulty breathing? yes. Tell me more about this.
has hay fever, some discomfort during attacks Takes Dristan

Do you have a cough? no Describe

Do you use tobacco? not now How much? What form?

Do you have any heart trouble? yes Describe heart attack 4 years ago

Any swollen or discolored parts of your body? no Describe

What time of day do you have your meals? 7[30], 1, 6[30] Snacks? no

What do you usually eat for

Breakfast?	Noon Meal?	Evening Meal?	Snacks?
plain toast orange juice cereal - milk coffee 1c.	meat green salad potato or rice vegetable fruit	sandwich soup fruit coffee 1c	

What foods or drinks do you dislike? fatty, oily foods, cream, mayonnaise

What foods or drinks do you like? most - Likes to eat one food at a time
Uses salt liberally

Do you need any help with eating? no Describe

Have you been on a special diet? no Describe

Estimate the number of glasses (cups) of fluid you drink each day.
Drinks a gallon of water a day in hot weather.

Do you have any trouble urinating? no Describe

How many times do you get up at night to urinate?

How often do your bowels move? 2 x a day What time of day? around 8 am, 9 pm.

Do you have constipation? no Diarrhea? no

What do you do to treat constipation? Diarrhea?

What time do you usually retire? 11[30] pm. Arise? 6[30] am

What routines do you go through in preparing for bed? shower

Figure 3.2. Nursing History: Interview Schedule

Do you have any trouble sleeping? no Describe

Says he requires only 6 hours sleep.

Has anything helped you to sleep better?

Do you take naps during the day? What time?

What do you usually do for exercise? bicycle. chop wood

How often do you do this? 2 - 3 times per week

How much exercise is involved in your usual day? In and out of car many times.

Are you right/left handed? right

Do you ever have chills? no Fever? no Night sweats? no

What brings them on?

Do you ever feel faint or light-headed? no Describe

Do you ever have pain or other discomfort? in chest Describe

"heart just exploded"

What brings it on? don't know What do you do for relief? Came to Emergency Room.

What kind of bath do you prefer? shower What time of day? 11 pm.

When do you brush your teeth? after breakfast & after evening meal

What brand of dentifrice do you prefer? Colgate's Mouthwash? none

Do you have dentures, bridgework? no What do you use for cleaning?

Do you have any skin problems? What skin preparations (soap, lotion) do you use? Shaves every morning.

Do you have any problems with seeing? Some Hearing? no Speaking? no

Describe wears glasses to drive car

Do you wear glasses? part time Contact lenses? Hearing aid?

What other languages do you speak? English

What do you like to do to keep in touch with relatives and friends?

visit, phone

Which church do you attend? First Baptist

Would you describe yourself as active, passive, or regularly attends regarding church?

What devotional literature do you usually read? New English Bible

If you wish your clergyman to visit you, what is his name? Rev R. J.

Do you have religious beliefs we should consider in planning your care?

Describe none

What do you do for recreation? bicycle with daughter Hobbies? Coin collecting

What would you like to do for diversion while ill? radio - T.V.

What is your occupation? water - meter reader

Figure 3.2. (Continued)

What are your usual working hours? 8 - 5

What are your feelings about your work? enjoys

When you become ill, whose help do you seek first? Dr. A. T.

When a physician prescribes a treatment, diet or medication for you, how closely do you follow his instructions? Fairly well - Gave up smoking after first M.I.

Do you have regular medical and dental checkups? no How often? ____

What do you do when you face a particularly stressful experience? he tries to think through best way to handle it.

What do you do when you are upset? go outside and work it off.

Whose counsel do you seek? wife, or pastor

COMPETENCIES: (From your contact with the patient, estimate his competencies.)

Physical other than heart attack, appears in good health for age.

Mental alert. Has adequate understanding of condition, and wants to learn more, so he can prevent another attack.

Emotional appears anxious and frightened, restless. Dreads period of inactivity enforced because of M.I.

Spiritual regularly attends church. Pastor knows he is in hospital and will visit.

Social worried about losing his job because of illness and because he has only one year until retirement.

Environment Home is one level. Wife drives. Telephone.

Wife and daughter are concerned, appear competent to carry on at home. Mrs. C. is a clerk in a food market, will continue to work and visit Mr C. in afternoon and evening.

Figure 3.2. (Concluded)

(The nursing care plan based on this nursing history may be found on page 98)

a more thorough nursing history than would a nurse with less experience or education.

Whether the history is recorded in outline form or essay form is determined by the preference of the nurse and by the policy of the agency. More important than format is the ready availability of the information for use in planning patient care. It may be helpful to underline or star those parts of the nursing history which are most significant in planning care. If an incomplete history is obtained, a list of information still needed should be included as a notation at the end of the write-up to serve as a reminder for those involved in the care of the patient.

To facilitate the recording of a nursing history in writing, an agency might well provide some type of dictating equipment so that the history can be transcribed in typewritten form by a secretarial assistant. Most nurses probably feel unprepared to use dictating machines, but an orientation to techniques of dictating could prepare them for this time-saving procedure. The saving of time, improved legibility, and consistent format for the nursing history might be worth the effort and expense.

* * * * *

The nursing history is obtained from an interview with the patient and/or his family at the initial encounter with the nurse for the current health/illness experience. The content of the nursing history and the methods for obtaining it vary according to the agency in which the nurse practices and the nature of the patient's health problem.

CLINICAL INSPECTION

When the nurse first sees the patient, she, in addition to obtaining the nursing history, assesses his physical status. Information from this clinical inspection gives the nurse a baseline from which she can observe change. The nurse will develop a systematic way of performing this inspection, but it should be flexible enough to allow for adjustments in her approach to various patients. A systematic approach tends to provide a framework so that important details are not overlooked. It tends to save time and be more efficient in terms of work organization.

Perhaps the most significant clues to the physical status of the patient are his vital signs and state of awareness. These measures, along with height and weight measurement, are a logical beginning for the clinical inspection.

One way of systematically inspecting a person is to begin at the head and proceed toward the toes, front to back. Another way is to use the physiological systems as a guide for inspection. A listing of items for clinical inspection patterned after the nursing history presented in Figure 3.3 of this chapter is included in the Summary of Assessment Data, pages 57-62. It is suggested that the clinical inspection follow the major areas of assessment: reactions, patterns of functioning, competencies.

Since there are a number of ways of doing a systematic clinical inspection, the nurse should select a way that is meaningful and efficient for her. The clinical inspection should note normal as well as abnormal findings, the presence or absence of conditions. Of particular interest to the nurse is the condition of the patient's integument, since the care of skin, hair, and nails is traditionally the responsibility of the nurse. Therefore she should

NURSING HISTORY

Semistructured Interview

Mr. A. B.

REACTIONS AND EXPECTATIONS

Present Health Problem aware that he is unable to move legs. Hopes surgery will restore movement. Wife and parents aware of probable prognosis - paraplegia

Past Health Problems
Has been in good health all his life. Only previous hospitalization was for T & A at 8 yrs. Remembers the ice cream and separation from parents.

Diagnostic Tests, Therapy, Rehabilitation
Has had limited experience. Does not know what to expect. Mrs. B. says he usually wants to know what is going on and why.

PATTERNS OF FUNCTIONING

Respiration
No problem. Does not smoke No known allergies. Multiple rib fractures, rt side - from accident.

Circulation
No problem

Food and Fluid Intake Drinks 10-12 cups of liquids per day. Enjoys food. Appears a little overweight. Is 5'11", weighs 185 lbs. Dislikes turnips and shellfish.

Breakfast 7am	Noon Meal 12³⁰ p.	Evening Meal 6³⁰ pm.	Snacks
1-2 fried eggs bacon or ham 2-3 slices toast orange juice or fruit 2-3 c. coffee.	2 sandwiches with salad or french fries 4-6 cookies apple or orange 2-3 c. coffee	meat potatoes cooked vegetable raw salad pie, cake or ice cream coffee	2-3 beers during evening.

Figure 3.3. Nursing History: Semistructured Interview

Elimination

No problems voiding. Does not get up at night
B.M. daily after breakfast, no straining

Rest/Sleep

Sleeps well. Goes to bed between 10 & 11 pm, up at 6^{30} a.m. Uses one pillow, 1-2 blankets, prefers cool, dark room. Takes shower before going to bed.

Exercise

Gets a lot of exercise as a truck driver, hauling produce. Also does weight-lifting almost every day.

Pain/Discomfort

Rarely has any pain. For an occasional headache takes Bufferin, tabs ii

Regulatory Mechanisms

No problems
Has always prided himself on control of his body. Satisfactory marital relationships.

Personal Hygiene

Showers @ H.S. Brushes teeth with Crest after breakfast and before going to bed. Washes hair once a week.

Communication

Is sedated now, but is coherent, uses English well. No problems seeing, hearing, speaking. Does not wear glasses.

Coping Patterns

"Sounds off" when he is upset - also does strenuous exercise. Usually looks at life realistically

Religious Life

Has never had a church affiliation.
No objection to chaplain visits

Social/Occupational Life

Husband and father. Proud of family - 4 children. Close-knit family & does things together. Truck driver. Belongs to Teamster's Union, not active in Union affairs

Figure 3.3. (Continued)

Recreation/Diversion
Jeeping around desert is favorite pastime. Belongs to a jeep club. Sustained present injury in jeep accident. Does own mechanical work on jeep. Watches news on T.V. & a few programs. Reads paper daily; little else.

Health Supervision
Sees family doctor only when one of family is ill. Dental check up annually.

COMPETENCIES

Physical Compression fracture & probable severed cord T10-11. Paralyzed distal to T10. Multiple rib fractures right side. Otherwise appears healthy c̄ strong, muscular build. Candidate for pulmonary complications, pressure sores, contractures. Will probably need bowel & bladder training, & wheel chair activity.

Mental
alert. High school education.

Emotional Usually faces problems realistically. When angry or upset reacts verbally & by physical exertion. Soon regains composure. May need to learn new ways of coping.

Spiritual
Has no church affiliation. Willing to have chaplain visit. Chaplain may be able to help with emotional adjustment to disability.

Social No vocational skills other than Truck driver. Union insurance will cover expenses for a while. Check if Union will help with Vocational Rehabilitation. Will probably need vocational counselling.

Environment
Home is 200 miles from Medical Center. Will need to find out about rehab. services nearer home. Home is one level, 2-3 steps to both outside doors. Yard is level. Find out how much wife can help with care.

N.B. Will re-assess post op. & begin active rehab. program as soon as possible after decompression laminectomy. May need to change dietary habits when less active. Will need to develop approach for helping him accept his disability.

Figure 3.3. (Concluded)

(The nursing care plan based on this nursing history may be found on page 100) describe the size, anatomical location, and appearance of all lesions. She should note the presence and extent of edema. If there are no lesions or edema, this is significant enough to be recorded. Her inspection should include the condition of oral mucosa, muscle tone, range of joint motion, breath sounds. While these latter items are also part of the physician's examination, the nurse must look and listen for herself if she is to have adequate information to establish a baseline. People may differ in describing such observations as color, sound, moisture. The nature, extent, and duration of all clinical signs and symptoms being experienced by the patient should be ascertained. Some of this information on signs and symptoms may be obtained from the physician's history and physical examination if they are written in unambiguous terms and contain the type of information the nurse needs to know.

The clinical inspection should include an assessment of the patient's functioning in relation to his age. Infants and children as well as adolescents and adults should be observed for physical and behavioral evidence of normal growth and development. Part of the nurse's knowledge essential for a clinical inspection includes an understanding of the developmental tools and tasks for each stage of life. From her assessment, the nurse should be able to determine a person's competencies in terms of his age.

Tools the nurse may use for a clinical inspection include a stethoscope, sphygmomanometer, clinical thermometer, tape measure, scales, timepiece, and possibly a flashlight and tongue depressor. A protractor-type goniometer can be useful in measuring any limitation of joint motion. For assessing a young child's development, certain toys and other objects may be used to test his coordination, physical and mental development. A Snellen eye chart or an audiometer are sometimes used by nurses. Nurses practicing in some settings or in an extended role (see Chapter 1) may use more complex equipment for clinical inspection of the patient than nurses customarily use. The most important tools a nurse uses are her own senses — eyes that see, ears that hear, hands that feel, a nose which detects odors, and a mind that understands.

Since a careful clinical inspection serves as a baseline from which to observe change, it is important to share this information so that all who care for the patient will recognize change. Therefore an accurate recording of all observations is essential. The descriptions of observations should be written in unambiguous terms, as objectively as possible regarding size, shape, color, texture, appearance, amount, anatomical location.

* * * * * *

A number of other assessment guides have been developed by nurses. These assessment guides may be used for nursing history, clinical inspection, and/or ongoing appraisal. Some of these guides are found in the sources listed below.[5-10]

ON-GOING APPRAISAL

As the patient progresses or regresses, his needs for nursing care will change. Because of these changes, the nurse must do regular reappraisals of his condition so that the care she plans will meet his needs. How often these reappraisals are done is usually determined by the lability of the patient's condition. For instance, a critically ill patient may need a partial appraisal every few minutes, whereas a long-term patient whose condition is stable may need reassessing at infrequent intervals – weekly, monthly, or at such times as new treatments or other developments occur.

The on-going appraisal consists of selected components from the nursing history and clinical inspection which indicate change from the baseline established on admission or at the beginning of some form of therapy. The particular items to be appraised will vary with each individual and will be determined by his clinical status, emotional reactions, attitudes, behavior, disease process, and medical prescription.

The nurse must select the components of the on-going appraisal which are important indicators of change or which were shown to be significant when the baseline was established. If a patient has no evidence of pressure areas on admission and is not confined to bed, there is little need to continue to check him for pressure sores. If a patient's blood pressure and other vital signs are stable, these may need checking only once or twice daily or even at less frequent intervals. If he goes to surgery, reacts to a medication, or develops some untoward symptoms, the frequency of checking his vital signs should be increased according to the severity of the changes and the precipitating condition. As his condition stabilizes, the frequency of checks can be lessened. Certain facts about the patient's disease process or treatment should prompt the nurse to appraise the patient for appropriate determinants of his condition. The patient with heart, liver, or kidney disease is very likely to develop edema, so he should

---

[5]Virginia Henderson, *Nature of Nursing* (New York: The Macmillan Company, 1966), p. 49.

[6]Faye G. Abdellah, *et al., Patient-Centered Approaches to Nursing* (New York: The Macmillan Company, 1960), pp. 16-17.

[7]R. Faye McCain, "Nursing by Assessment – not Intuition," *American Journal of Nursing* 65:4(1965):82-84.

[8]Doris A. Geitgey, "Self-Pacing – A Guide to Nursing Care," *Nursing Outlook* 17:8(1969):48-49.

[9]Virginia Apgar, *et al.*, "Evaluation of the Newborn Infant – Second Report," *Journal of the American Medical Association* 168:15(1958):1985-1988.

[10]Freeman and Lowe, "A Method for Appraising Family Public Health Nursing Needs."

be weighed periodically, his fluid intake and output measured. Likewise, the effectiveness of diuretic therapy or a restricted sodium diet can be ascertained by measuring intake, output, and body weight. Most surgical patients have an inhibition of peristalsis for a period of time after surgery, so the on-going appraisal should include checks for abdominal distention, "gas pains," and passage of flatus.

Physical and emotional status of the patient may indicate the possibility of certain complications. With these possible complications in mind, the nurse should include in her on-going appraisal observations indicating the early development of these complications. She would initiate nursing measures to prevent these complications insofar as possible. The absence of any signs that the complications were occurring would be a reliable evaluation of her preventive nursing measures. It is particularly important for nurses caring for patients confined to bed to be thoroughly familiar with the hazards of bedrest. This knowledge should prompt the nurse to initiate preventive measures and to regularly appraise the patient for early signs of these complications.[11]

Part of the nurse's on-going assessment is a look at the patient's needs for general care in terms of his place on the dependency-independency continuum. In other words, what can the patient do for himself and with what does he need help? How much help does he require? What can he do today that he could not do yesterday? All aspects of personal hygiene, exercise, posture, eating, drinking, and eliminating should be reviewed to determine the patient's needs for help and what he can or should do for himself. Also considered on the dependency scale are the patient's physical and emotional status and his needs for instruction and counseling since he is dependent on the nurse for these needs.

Several guides have been created for categorizing patients according to their dependency or to the acuity of their needs for nursing care. Most of these are adaptations of a scheme originated by the United States Army. A task force appointed by the California Nurses' Association[12] adapted and enlarged the army plan to a workable definition of categories. Each category includes a list of typical symptoms, treatments, observation or instruction measures needed, methods of controlling activity, and deviations from acceptable behavior patterns. These categories are used to classify patients according to their needs. The task force stated unequivocally that the professional nurse practitioner is the only one who has the knowledge, judgment, and values necessary for assessing the kind

---

[11] Edith V. Olson, et al., "The Hazards of Immobility," *American Journal of Nursing* 67:4(1967):779-797.

[12] Lauraine A. Thomas, Chairman, Task Force IV, *Establishing Staffing Patterns Based on Acuity of Patient Needs,* (San Francisco, California, Nurses' Association, November, 1968).

and degree of nursing needs of the individual patient. If the patient's dependency status is a meaningful assessment, it must be included in the on-going appraisal and must be done periodically according to the patient's changing needs.

Assessment needed for discharge planning should begin when a patient is admitted to a facility. However, many circumstances may preclude gathering the necessary information at the time of admission. If this information was not obtained or if it was incomplete, the nurse should obtain the necessary information as soon as circumstances permit. Assessment data necessary for discharge planning include information regarding the patient, the family, and the facility to which the patient will be going, whether to his home or to another health care agency.

A careful estimate of the patient's competencies in all the components of wholeness is particularly important for discharge planning. Some questions for which answers will be needed include:

What will be his dependency level?

In what particular functions of daily living will the patient be independent? With which functions will he need help?

What does the patient need to learn about self care, about accepting help, and about community resources?

Who will be available to help the patient? How competent are these helping people? What do they need to be taught?

Is the environment to which the patient is going healthful and safe?

Are there environmental factors which could be deleterious to the patient?

What adjustments in home, transportation, other areas, will be necessary to accommodate for the patient's disability?

In what ways will the care of the patient affect his family? What help do they need to prepare for his discharge?

What community agencies can assist the patient? Which agencies has he used in the past?

The on-going appraisal of the patient should elicit information which can be used for discharge planning as well as for daily planning.

Tools used for on-going appraisal are the same as those used for clinical inspection. Interviewing skills are necessary for appraising attitudes and reactions and for determining levels of self-help. Several of the assessment guides mentioned in the preceding section are also useful guides for on-going appraisal of the patient's needs for nursing care.

The Summary of Assessment Data (pages 57-62) indicates some items for the on-going appraisal in terms of the patient's reactions to and expectations of his day-to-day therapy, changes in his patterns of functioning, and his levels of competency.

OTHER SOURCES

The Medical Record

From the reports of the medical history and physical examinations in the medical record, the nurse can note clues regarding the possible signs and symptoms that the patient might experience; there may be some clues for needed health teaching; and there will be a record of the patient's past illnesses and hospitalizations. The physician's plan of therapy for the patient may be ascertained. Knowing the medical diagnosis of the patient can give some indication of the probable course of the patient's health/illness experience and should help the nurse anticipate certain complications. Some of these complications might be prevented by nursing measures, so they should be considered when planning nursing care.

The medical record is also the source of those responsibilities for patient care delegated to the nurse by the physician. Ascertaining what these delegated treatments and observations are and how they fit into the patient's total regimen is essential to the planning of both nursing care and the team approach.

Progress notes recorded by the physician are a running account of the patient's responses to therapy. The progress record may confirm or deny the nurse's own observations, and it may explain some of her questions about the patient. Often, problems in patient care are presented in the progress notes, and the nurse should consider what nursing can do to help resolve these problems. Diagnostic and therapeutic procedures proposed by the physician should alert the nurse to prepare the patient for these experiences.

While the medical record is a rich source of information about the patient and his care, its use does not supplant face-to-face conferences with the physician regarding the care of the patient. The physician is the leader of the health team and, if the nurse is to fulfill her role as coordinator of the patient's care, there must be a close working relationship with the physician. It is essential to know what his aims and expectations are for the patient and how nursing can contribute to the attainment of these objectives.

Results of clinical laboratory and radiological examinations may provide clues to nursing problems presented by the patient as well as indicate the need for specific observations, health teaching, or therapeutic measures. For instance, a low hemoglobin may explain the patient's fatigue, may indicate the need for a more careful diet history, and may lead to teaching regarding dietary change if diet is the cause of his low hemoglobin. An increasing serum bilirubin should alert the nurse to observe color changes in skin and sclera, urine and stools, and may lead to her consulting with the physician regarding the need for isolation, dietary changes, and a program of rest. The effects of high serum bilirubin on the central nervous system give rise to a need for careful observation and recording of the patient's state of awareness. Pruritis may also develop and signal the need for special skin care. Even though the nurse should note these signs and symptoms without knowledge of the laboratory examination, the knowledge should increase her awareness and also should broaden her perspective of nursing care. A decreasing white blood cell count accompanying certain forms of drug therapy should provide the clue to initiate protective isolation of the patient. Chest X-ray reports are helpful in specifying positions for postural drainage. The nurse might be less likely to get the information in the two preceding instances without the reports.

The Literature

Only as a nurse continues to learn in conjunction with her practice of nursing is she truly a professional person. The problems presented by patients are numerous and varied and no one can learn enough in his educational program to provide solutions to the many nursing problems encountered in clinical practice. By keeping abreast of current literature, the nurse can increase her expertise in problem identification and she is more likely to suggest innovative solutions to problems. From her reading the nurse may learn about new approaches to common problems and may gain greater insight and understanding of these.

When presented with a patient problem with which the nurse is unprepared to cope, she should not hesitate to do library research on the topic in order to gain the knowledge necessary to plan the nursing care of the patient. Unique and unusual situations in the practice of her profession should induce the nurse to refer to the literature in order to know how to cope with the situations and to plan appropriate nursing care. However, the challenge of the unique and unusual must not overshadow nor dull the challenge of the commonplace. The common problems of patients often lull the nurse into routinized, stereotyped forms of nursing care not personalized to the patient. Such nursing practice soon deteriorates to a low level, and the nurse's satisfaction with her job will soon fall to a low level also.

To keep up with new drugs, diagnostic measures, and therapies is a tremendous task, but the nurse cannot limit herself to the medical aspects of these new developments. More important is to ascertain the implications for nursing observations and nursing care arising from these new drugs and techniques.

Nursing is as broad as life since it deals with people, so the nurse's reading should give her a broader and deeper understanding of human beings — their culture as well as their physiology, their social problems as well as their disease processes, their emotional and spiritual nature as well as their biological functioning.

Unless a nurse is constantly challenged to find creative and innovative solutions to both common and unusual nursing problems, she cannot function on a high professional plane. This challenge must come from within; it cannot be imposed by an external force. It requires commitment to the profession of nursing and a growing respect and concern for the persons she serves. The price is high; the rewards are great. The rewards are not measured in dollars and cents but in personal satisfaction and a deep sense of having contributed to the health and happiness of human beings.

The Social History

The social history may give the nurse clues regarding the patient's home situation, occupational problems, economic worries, and interpersonal relationships. Information from the social history may explain some of the patient's concerns, may indicate a need for early discharge planning, and may show what referrals have been made and disclose the need for other referrals.

Some clues as to cultural, religious, or economic constraints imposed upon the individual or family may be revealed by the social history. Social histories may reveal more about the family structure than the nurse obtained in her history, may itemize the strengths and weaknesses of the family. It may also be the source of important information about the home and the community in which the patient resides. This information may be useful to the nurse in identifying problems, in suggesting a need for referrals, in pointing out a need for health teaching, and in implying a need for team approach to discharge planning. This information is vital to developing the total plan of patient care.

The nurse uses a variety of sources of data about the patient and/or family for whom she is caring. Some data come from the patient, the family, or other health personnel and from the literature. All are necessary to the planning of personalized nursing care. When these data are sorted into various categories, it is possible to identify the nursing problems of the patient and/or family.

Table 3.1
Summary of Assessment Data

Nursing History	*Clinical Inspection*	*On-going Appraisal*	*Other Sources*
REACTIONS AND EXPECTATIONS			
Present Illness			
Meaning of illness to patient, family. How illness interfered with life. Understandings re: nature of illness, plan of care. Feelings about hospitalization. What would you like to know about tests and treatments planned? What would you like to know about the results of tests and treatments? What effect do you expect this illness to have on your life? Do you expect any change in ability to function as a man? husband? father? woman? wife? mother? Attitudes toward body exposure for examination and treatments (modesty).	Facial expression Mannerisms Muscle tension Evidence of skin reactions	Feelings re: day's program? new regimen? Expectations re: diagnostic tests, diet? medication? other therapy? rehabilitation program? dismissal? transfer? labor and delivery? Reactions to alterations in body image. Position on dependency scale. Reactions to dependency. Reactions to separation from family or usual life situation.	Social history may include effects of illness on family. Medical history may include some reactions to present illness, past therapy. Medical examination and progress notes may include reactions to tests, treatments.
Previous Illness			
What experiences have you had in hospitals (agencies) before? What did you like about the nursing care? Dislike? Reactions to previous separation from family.			Medical history will list causes of previous hospitalizations and nature of past illnesses. May list immunizations.
PATTERNS OF FUNCTIONING		**For each function:** Select from observations listed in clinical inspection those appropriate to patient's condition. Note changes from base line established with history and clinical inspection. Note symptoms related to each function. Note behavior accompanying symptom – especially with small children and nonverbal adults. Frequency of observation depends on clinical problem.	**For each function:** Medical diagnosis, surgery, medication or other therapy or diagnostic tests affecting the function. Are there complications or emergencies arising from the health/illness problem which could affect the function? What can nursing do to prevent them?

Table 3.1. (*Continued*)

Nursing History	*Clinical Inspection*	*On-going Appraisal*	*Other Sources*
		In what way has disease process or type of therapy altered usual pattern of functioning? Assess need for teaching or counseling re: therapy, rehabilitation, prevention, or change in pattern.	
Respiration			
Ever feel out of breath? What brings this on? Effect of position, exercise on breathing? Cough? Productive? Frequency of cough? Does cough interfere with rest? Sneeze? When? What brings it on? Regularly do breathing exercises? Describe. Use tobacco? form? amount?	Rate, rhythm, symmetry, depth, effort of breathing, use of accessory muscles, splinting? Contour of chest. Breath sounds. Rales? Nature and depth of cough. Appearance of sputum. Vital capacity? Tidal volume.	Dyspnea, orthopnea, amount and appearance of secretions. Tracheostomy – secretions, condition of stoma.	Results of pulmonary function studies, blood gas studies, chest X-rays.
Circulation			
Does your heart pound? Skip beats? What brings this on? What do you do to relieve this? Any parts of body feel colder or warmer than adjacent parts? Any discolored parts? Any swollen, edematous areas?	Pulse rate, rhythm, quality, apical/radial rates, pulse deficit. Quality and presence of peripheral pulses. Electrocardiogram or oscilloscope pattern. Blood pressure, pulse pressure, central venous pressure, arterial mean pressure. Temperature, color of body parts, especially extremities, ears, lips. Edema? pitting? where? extent? Circumference of edematous extremities. Capillary refilling time. Pressure areas? Any inflamed areas.	Arrhythmias. Interference with circulation to a part. Hemorrhage.	Interpretation of ECG and other tests of heart function, angiograms, etc. Hematology. Blood chemistry.
Food and Fluid Intake			
Number and times of meals, snacks. Usual content of breakfast, noon meal, evening meal, snacks. Amount of coffee, tea, beer, liquor, other beverages per day. Likes and dislikes in food and beverages. Amount and kind of oils, fats, cream, spreads? Amount and kinds of seasoning.	Weight, height, body build. Hydration of mucous membranes. Nutritional status of skin, scalp, nails. Color and texture of skin.	Appetite. Actual food, fluids taken. Does therapy interfere with food or fluid intake? Type and rate of intravenous infusion or other parenteral feeding. Relation of intake to output. Results of tests for urine sugar, acetone, pH.	Allergies. Results of G.I. tract X-rays and other studies, liver function tests, blood-sugar levels. Prescription re: diet, fluids.

Table 3.1. (*Continued*)

Nursing History	*Clinical Inspection*	*On-going Appraisal*	*Other Sources*
Stability of weight? Recent gain or loss? Cause known?		Acceptance of therapeutic diet.	
When was last meal?			
Extent of help required with eating.			
Frequency, type, and amount of infant's feeding.			
Food groups: number of servings of milk products? meat, eggs, cheese? fruits and vegetables? breads and cereals?			
Elimination			
Frequency of voiding? day? night? urgency?		Frequency, amount and appearance of urine, feces, perspiration.	Results of barium enema, stools studies, kidney function tests, blood chemistry, urinalysis.
Frequency and time of bowel movement.		Contour of abdomen.	
Use of enemas? laxatives? suppositories?		Passage of flatus.	
		Catheter function.	
If an 'ostomy, how do you manage?	Appearance of stoma. Type of appliance used.	Need for laxative, etc.	
Words used by child re: elimination.		Acceptance of 'ostomy.	
Degree of child's independence in toileting.			
Rest and Sleep			
Average number of hours of sleep?		Actual hours slept.	Check medical record for rest prescription.
Time of retiring? arising? What done in preparation for bed?		Nature of rest, sleep.	
		Acceptance of rest regimen.	
		Need for sedation.	
Feelings on arising?		Need for teaching re: rest, relaxation, sleep habits.	
Any difficulty getting to sleep? staying asleep?			
What helps you sleep?			
What interferes with sleep? (light, noise, etc.)			
Preferred kind and amount of bedding.			
Number of pillows.			
Sleeping room warm? cool?			
Daytime rest periods? naps?			
Favorite toy or blanket for child?			
Exercises			
What usually done for exercise? frequency? amount?	Extent of range of joint motion.		Items in clinical inspection column may be included in physician's physical examination.
How much walking per day?	Muscle tonus, atrophy, turgor.		Check Physical Medicine evaluation.
	Posture.		
Activity involved in usual day?	Gait.		

Table 3.1. (*Continued*)

Nursing History	*Clinical Inspection*	*On-going Appraisal*	*Other Sources*
Right- or left-handed? Steps, stairs in home? place of work?	Prosthetic devices.	Need for teaching re: exercise habits, posture, gait.	
Pain/Discomfort			
Pain or discomfort frequently experienced? Describe. What done to relieve? Feelings (concerns) re: above pain/discomfort. Cause known? What would like nurses to do to relieve pain/discomfort?	Describe physical manifestations of pain or discomfort present.	Nature, duration, extent of pain or other discomfort. Evaluation of relief measures. Muscle guarding due to pain. Is pain/discomfort following expected pattern?	Check physician's record for symptoms of which patient complains.
Regulatory Mechanisms			
Chills? fever? perspire profusely? tolerance of heat? cold? Fainting? dizzy spells? seizures? Menstruation – when due? supplies needed? Menopause? hot flashes? Hormone replacement therapy? Birth control pills?	Temperature: oral, axillary, or rectal. Signs of infection. Moisture and color of skin. Tics, paralysis. State of awareness—level of consciousness. Response to stimuli—tactile, verbal, pressure, thermal, painful. Tests and questions to see if development consistent with age.	Need for teaching or counseling re: menstrual hygiene, contraception, etc.	Check medical history and physical examination for neurological tests. Hormone therapy. Results of hormone studies, CNS X-rays and other studies.
Perinatal patient: Onset of contractions. When is baby due? Have membranes ruptured?	Frequency and duration of contractions. Intact membranes? Vaginal bleeding?	Behavioral and physiological changes consistent with stage of labor. Height and firmness of fundus. Amount and appearance of lochia. Breast engorgement, tenderness, state of nipples. Appearance of perineal area. Need for teaching re: postnatal care or infant care.	Pregnancy record.
Personal Hygiene			
Kind, time, frequency of bath, shampoo? Oral hygiene – time, frequency? Preferred dentifrice, mouthwash? Denture care? Nail, cutical problem? What done for any skin conditions? Frequency and time of shaving.	Condition of skin, scalp, hair, nails, mouth.	Ability for self-care. Need for teaching re: personal hygiene.	

Table 3.1. (*Continued*)

Nursing History	*Clinical Inspection*	*On-going Appraisal*	*Other Sources*
Communication and Special Senses			
Any difficulty speaking, hearing, seeing, understanding English? read, write English?	Manner of speaking, tone of voice. Words, tone of voice consistent with affect.		Results of sight, hearing tests.
What done to keep in touch with family, friends, business?	Mannerisms. Coherence of expressions.		
What name does child or adolescent prefer?	Presence of glasses, contact lenses, hearing aid, speech defect.		
Coping with Stress			
What done when facing stressful situations?	Attitudes, moods.	Coping mechanisms observed during stressful circumstances.	Results of psychiatric evaluation.
Whose advice sought?		Need to learn better ways of coping.	
What do you do when you are upset? angry? frightened?		Attitude toward change. Postnatal patients: Response to motherhood. Ways of handling baby. Concerns re: baby's body. Remarks re: infant's characteristics	
Religious Life			
Usual pattern of worship, church attendance?	Religious medals worn.	Ability to meet own spiritual needs.	Chaplain or clergyman.
Active/passive participant.			
Type of personal devotions, religious literature read.			
Wish clergyman to visit? who?		Need for religious counselor.	
Religious beliefs and practices re: diet, day of worship, holy days, birth, death, blood transfusion, use of drugs.			
Social/Occupational Life			
Work role—type and hours of work. Feelings re: work.		Response to visitors, phone calls, mail.	Check social history re: social, occupational problems.
Family roles.		Support of family, friends.	
Members of household.		Behavior toward roommates, visitors, staff.	
Social roles—kinds of social activities of interest.		Acceptance of sick role or other role change.	
Will family/friends be able to visit?		Need for teaching and counseling re: vocational rehabilitation.	
Any especially want to see? not want to see?			
Cultural prescriptions re: health care and practices.			
Recreation/Diversion			
What done for fun? hobby? vacation?		Evidence of boredom?	
What to do to pass time while ill?			

Table 3.1. (*Concluded*)

Nursing History	*Clinical Inspection*	*On-going Appraisal*	*Other Sources*
Have interests you would like to pursue but never had the time?			
Child's favored play activities and playthings.			
Health Supervision			
When physician prescribes a special diet, medication, or program, how closely do you follow it?			Medical history may include past practices re: seeking and following medical advice.
What kinds of illness send you to bed?			
What reasons do you stay off work?		Need for teaching or counseling, re: self-medication, health supervision, use of community facilities.	
For what reasons do you consult a doctor? dentist?			
Whose help do you seek first when you become ill?		Need for planning with patient or family re: home care or transfer to another facility.	
What community agencies have you used in the past? for what purpose?			
Keep appointments?			
Yearly examination?			
What immunizations have you had? when?			
Who can help with your care when you return home?			

COMPETENCIES

Physical

General status of health; dependence on others, drugs prostheses, or other measures; ability to carry out prescription, preventive measures, therapeutic regimen, or rehabilitation program.

Mental

Ability to understand, to relate cause to effect, to solve problems, to communicate with others, to recall near and distant events; educational (language) background.

Emotional

Maturity; make and carry out decisions; responsibility for own behavior.

Spiritual

Strength of religious faith, dependence on faith or religion in everyday life or crises.

Social

Family integrity, respect, support, and love given and received. Sharing of responsibility, quality of performance of work, social and family roles; income and insurance sufficient for needs.

Environment

Available health services; safety, space, and privacy of home; suitability of home in relation to disability; transportation, telephone, chemical and bacteriologic problems in home or work environment. Environmental hazards which might aggravate health/illness problems.

REFERENCES

ABDELLAH, FAYE G. *et al. Patient Centered Approaches to Nursing.* New York: The Macmillan Co., 1960, pp. 1-19.

APGAR, VIRGINIA. "Evaluation of the Newborn Infant—Second Report." *Journal of the American Medical Association* 168:15(1958):1985-8.

*BYERS, VIRGINIA B. *Nursing Observation.* Dubuque, Iowa: Wm. C. Brown Company Publishers, 1968.

CHRISTENSEN, KATHRYN A., and KILEY, MARYLOU. "The Public Health Nurse and the Long-Term Neurologic Patient." *Nursing Clinics of North America* 4:2(1969):275-83.

*DAHLIN, BERNICE. "Rehabilitation and the Assessment of Patient Need." *Nursing Clinics of North America* 1:3(1966):375-86.

*FREEMAN, RUTH B. and LOWE, MARIE. "A Method for Appraising Family Public Health Nursing Needs." *American Journal of Public Health* 53:1 (1963):47-52.

*GEITGEY, DORIS A. "Self-Pacing—A Guide to Nursing Care." *Nursing Outlook* 17:8(1969):48-9.

GENTRY, ELIZABETH, and PARIS, LULU MAE. "Tools to Evaluate Child Development." *American Journal of Nursing* 67:12(1967):2544-6.

*GILBO, DONA. "Nursing Assessment of Circulatory Function." *Nursing Clinics of North America* 3:1(1968):53-63.

*HAMILTON, CONSTANCE B., *et al.* "The Nurse's Active Role in Assessment." *Nursing Clinics of North America* 4:2(1969):249-62.

HENDERSON, VIRGINIA. *The Nature of Nursing.* New York: The Macmillan Co., 1966.

KATONA, ELIZABETH A. "A Patient-Centered Living-Oriented Approach to the Patient With an Artificial Anus or Bladder." *Nursing Clinics of North America* 2:4(1967):623-34.

*KURIHARA, MARIE. "Assessment and Maintenance of Adequate Respiration." *Nursing Clinics of North America* 3:1(1968):65-76.

*MANTHEY, MARIE E. "A Guide for Interviewing." *American Journal of Nursing* 67:10(1967):2088-90.

*MCCAIN, R. FAYE. "Nursing by Assessment—not Intuition," *American Journal of Nursing* 65:4(1965):82-4.

*MCPHETRIDGE, L. MAE. "Nursing History: One Means to Personalize Care." *American Journal of Nursing* 68:1(1968)68-75.

*MINCKLEY, BARBARA B. "The Multiphasic Human-to-Human Monitor." *Nursing Clinics of North America* 3:1(1968)29-39.

*MODELL, WALTER, *et al. Handbook of Cardiology for Nurses.* New York: Springer Publishing Co., 1966, pp. 35-44.

OLSON, EDITH V., *et al.* "The Hazards of Immobility." *American Journal of Nursing* 67:4(1967):779-97.

*PAULUS, ALIXE C. "A Tool for the Assessment of the Retarded Child at Home. *Nursing Clinics of North America* 1:4(1966):659-68.

*RILEY, MILDRED. "The Nursing Interview for Psychiatric Patients." *Nursing Outlook* 16:10(1968):54-7.

SCHWARTZ, DORIS R. "Toward More Precise Evaluation of Patient's Needs." *Nursing Outlook* 13:5(1965):42-4.

*TRYON, PHYLLIS A. "Assessing the Progress of Labor Through Observation of Patient's Behavior." *Nursing Clinics of North America* 3:2(1968):315-26.

*Suggested for additional reading.

TRYON, PHYLLIS A. "Patient Participation vs Patient Passivity." *Nursing Forum.* II:2(1963):48-57.

TRYON, PHYLLIS A., and LEONARD, ROBERT C. "The Effect of the Patient's Participation on the Outcome of a Nursing Procedure." *Nursing Forum* III:2(1964):79-89.

YOUNG, JESSIE F. "Recognition, Significance, and Recording of the Signs of Increased Intracranial Pressure." *Nursing Clinics of North America* 4:2(1969):223-36.

CLINICAL EXPERIENCE

1. Select three patients of comparable clinical status. Use a different method of taking a nursing history (questionnaire, interview schedule, semistructured interview) on each patient and compare the quality of nursing histories.
2. Complete a nursing history and clinical inspection on a newly admitted patient. Use the data for developing a nursing care plan.
3. Compare a nursing history and a medical history on one patient and identify areas of overlap.
4. Compare nursing care plans based on a nursing history with those not based on a nursing history.

Chapter 4

Assessment—Problem Identification and Priority Setting

Once data have been collected and compiled in some organized fashion so that all pertaining to any one topic are together, these data can be analyzed to see what problems or needs the patient or family presents. In other words, data from the nursing history, clinical inspection, on-going appraisal, and other sources must all be classified in similar categories. Each category may be regarded as a problem area from which no problems or several may arise. If the classification of data is carried out as the information is gathered, both time and energy are saved.

To be consistent with the suggested assessment content presented in Chapter 3, all data concerning the patient's reactions and expectations, when reviewed, should indicate problematic reactions or unrealistic expectations. The data about each pattern of functioning should point out imbalances, unhealthful practices, or discomforts to be relieved. Data concerning the patient's various competencies denote strengths that can be built upon and weaknesses with which the person needs help. Of course, the data may also indicate several areas in which no significant problems exist.

ANALYSIS OF DATA

Data concerned with any one problem area must be examined to see whether a problem exists and to discover the nature of the problem which is presented. The information is reviewed for its meaning in terms of nursing care. It should be determined if the data point out a need which can be met in one way or another by the practice of nursing.

Regarding each set of data, the nurse might ask several questions. What is the relationship of the parts to the whole? to each other? What is the effect on the person's integrity and total well-being? Are effects appropriate to causes? Is there evidence of lack, excess, imbalance? Is there a need for change? What is the patient's potential in this area, and is his current status at or below this? Is there evidence of limitation, strength, weakness, dependency, independency? What adaptations are necessary because of the health/illness problem? Is there a possibility that a problem will occur unless some preventive action is implemented?

Some of the data will supply information which will help the nurse adapt her nursing care to the desires and usual daily patterns of the patient. Such data should not be used to "create" problems but should be used in constructing the nursing care plan. For example, the nursing history should indicate whether a patient prefers to brush his teeth before or after meals. This desire should be transmitted to the nursing care plan, but such data probably do not give a clue to a nursing problem. Perhaps another patient indicates that he prefers a certain type of diet because of his religious beliefs. This information is important in planning his care but does not point out a problem unless the diet is inadequate in essential nutrients or incompatible with the therapeutic diet. Much of the information regarding the patient's patterns of functioning will be of this type. If a disease process or the therapeutic program interferes with a pattern of functioning, one or more problems might be related to the affected patterns of functioning. When analyzing the data concerning the patient, it is important to recognize which data gives clues to nursing problems and which data are merely used to personalize the care of the patient. Following are some examples of patient data and the problem that was identified from the data.

Data: Mr. G. has an ileostomy.
He has lung abscesses with both tube and cutaneous drainage.
He has lost 60 pounds.
He has several recent incisions in his abdomen and chest.
Some of his statements include:
"I'm so thin," "I'm weak," "There's not much left of me,"
"My bones stick into the bed," "Now I have holes all over me."
With these statements, his tone of voice and facial expression show anger and disgust.

Problem: Unable to accept altered body image.

Data: Mr. H. has four or five episodes of coughing every hour.
He coughs up thick, purulent, yellow-brown material.
Mr. H. states he has a virus infection.
Chest x-ray shows an area of consolidation in left lower lobe.
Mr. H. says he cannot rest because of the cough.
Rest is one of Mr. H's prescribed therapies.

Problems: Cough interferes with rest.
Could cough be made more efficient?

Data: Mrs. I. says she is unable to sleep.
Mrs. I. says the monitor "beep" keeps her awake.
Mrs. I. reports discomfort at site of intravenous needle keeps her from relaxing.
Night nurse reports Mrs. I. awake at three different hourly checks.
Problem: Therapy interferes with sleep.

Data: Mrs. J. is on a 1000 calorie, 500 mg. sodium diet.
Mrs. J. picks at food on each tray, tastes each dish, rarely takes more than a taste.
Mrs. J. complains of being hungry.
Mrs. J. previously has salted her food before she tasted it.
Problem: Dislikes therapeutic diet.

Data: Mr. K. frequently talks about not being able to return to work.
His previous job was heavy manual labor.
Mr. K. has had a myocardial infarction.
Mr. K. reports that his physician says he can do some light work after four to six months.
Mrs. K. says she will get a job, Mr. K. does not approve.
Mr. K. appears despondent when he talks about working.
Mr. K. completed only seven grades in school, has done a variety of types of unskilled, hard work.
Problem: Conflict regarding dependency status and inability to return to former job.

NURSING PROBLEMS

Ability to identify nursing problems and solve them is an act of professional nursing. Nursing problems arise from difficulties experienced by a person or family within the context of health or illness.

Included in the dictionary definition of problem are these phrases: "a perplexing question, situation or person; a matter involving difficulty in solving, settling, or handling.'[1] A nursing problem then would be any perplexing health/illness situation faced by the person (or family), or any health/illness matter which the person (or family) has difficulty solving, settling, or handling with which the nurse can help. The type of help the nurse can give derives from the various roles of nursing and the three components of nursing: care, cure, and coordination (See Chapter 1).

Nursing problems arise when the person cannot meet his own needs, requires assistance with meeting a need, or is unable to cope with some phase of life. Problems also occur when a person is trying to meet needs in an inappropriate way or is not aware of a need. The data may indicate that the person has some discomfort which he is unable to relieve, lacks

[1]Webster's *New International Dictionary of the English Language,* 2nd ed. unabridged (Springfield, Massachusetts: G. C. Merriam Company, Publisher, 1961), p. 1971.

knowledge about some aspect of his program or of good health practices, is not motivated to function at his optimal level. On the other hand, the data may show that the patient is unable to accept some change in his usual life patterns, that he is having difficulty adapting to a disability or to a therapeutic regimen. Data may show an imbalance among the various components of wholeness. Other data may imply a need for the patient to work toward independence or interdependence in some aspect of living. Nursing problems may arise from inconsistencies between a person's potential and his actual level of living or between what he would like to be and what he is.

Data obtained by the nurse may point up problems largely outside the province of nursing – problems which are the concern of the physician, dietitian, social service worker, or some other member of the health-related professions. Data regarding problems outside of nursing may be of relevance to nursing insofar as the data help the nurse adapt care to the patient or as she refers the patient or family to a person who can help with the problem. Such data may indicate a need for continuing reappraisal of the problem by the nurse until others have accepted the problem for solution. For instance, a community health nurse may find a patient who presents all the symptoms of diabetes mellitus, yet she must refer the patient to a physician for diagnosis. She must continue to observe the patient and encourage him to seek medical attention. Once a medical diagnosis is made, the nurse will work with the patient on a different set of problems.

Sometimes the same problem is attacked in different ways by several different health professions; the differences are in terms of areas of emphasis or in types of solutions offered. To illustrate, a person may have insufficient money to supply food for himself and his family. The nurse may be concerned with the problem because the nutrition of the family is inadequate. She and/or a dietitian may teach them about low-cost meal planning and may recommend shopping techniques to stretch the food dollar. The nurse may refer the family to resources within the community who can provide economic assistance.

When data have been categorized under the patient's reactions and expectations, patterns of functioning and competencies as outlined in the Summary of Assessment Data (pages 57-62), certain problems will be pointed out. Some examples of nursing problems in each of these general areas follow.

Nursing problems arising from the patient's reactions to illness or hospitalization and his expectations regarding the outcome of his illness or of the services received include:

Does not know what to expect from diagnostic tests.
Conflict over role change from breadwinner to dependent person.
Unable to accept dependency.

Is afraid of anesthesia and surgery.
Unable to accept diagnosis of diabetes mellitus.
Expects radiation therapy to cure advanced malignancy.
Expects annual physical examinations for family of four to cost less than $50.00.

A nursing problem exists when a person's patterns of functioning are interfered with or cannot be maintained in the usual way, do not function normally, or are not conducive to optimal health. Some examples of this kind of problem are:

Constant abdominal pain.
Constipation.
Does not practice preventive oral hygiene.
Unable to relax and sleep sufficiently.
Bored with inactivity during hospitalization.
Insufficient milk included in family's diet.

A person's level of competency in any area may be a source of nursing problems. Examples of these problems include:

Insufficient funds for needed medical care.
Hard of hearing, no hearing aid.
Believes pain and disease are punishment for sins.
More dependent than physical status warrants.
Breathing problem aggravated by air pollution in home community.
Unable to manipulate insulin syringe because of arthritis.
Lacks transportation to hospital for daily physical therapy.

In the present status of nursing as a profession, there is little consensus regarding how nursing problems are stated. How the problem is stated is less important than the fact that the problem is identified and that nursing care is derived from it. The most important consideration in stating the problem is that the meaning and intent are communicated to those engaged in working with the problems – the patient and the nursing personnel. Some nurses prefer to think of patient needs rather than patient problems. Such thinking does not alter the process; it merely changes the wording so that a need is indicated rather than a problem. Whichever way is easier for the nurse to think through the nursing process, that method should be adopted. Nursing objectives and nursing care may be derived from either problems or needs.

Some attempts at developing a nomenclature for nursing problems have been made. Abdellah's twenty-one nursing problems[2] is an example. Several nursing texts have been written around Abdellah's classification, yet the classification has hardly met with unanimous acceptance. Some nurses regard the twenty-one statements as objectives rather than problems. Some of the categories seem to overlap and there is some ambiguity of meaning.

[2]Faye Abdellah, *et al.*, *Patient-Centered Approaches to Nursing* (New York: The Macmillan Company, 1960), page 19.

Overlapping is especially seen in the groups of emotional and interpersonal difficulties and community or social problems. This is a common shortcoming of most of the attempts to standardize nursing terms; the problem areas presented in this monograph are no exception.

The Twenty-One Problems have served as an incentive in directing nursing to the need for some standardization of terms. Indeed, it is time for the nursing profession to develop a standardized nomenclature of nursing problems or needs which conveys as much meaning among nurses as a diagnosis of congestive heart failure conveys among physicians.

* * * * *

After the problems or needs of the patient or family have been identified, they should be arranged in rank order of priority. This phase is necessary because some problems may be more crucial than others. It may not be possible to attempt solutions to all the problems presented. The setting of priorities may occur at different points of the nursing process. Not only must problems or needs be arranged in order of priority but also priorities must be determined for nursing objectives and nursing actions. Some criteria for determining priorities are applicable at any time when priorities must be set.

SETTING PRIORITIES

Priority refers to something that takes precedence over others in order of time or importance. It is concerned with putting first things first. It means choosing to do one thing and leaving something else undone or done later or not as well as desired. It may mean designing nursing care to solve some problems of the patient and leaving some problems unsolved. It may mean working on short-term goals because of their immediacy or urgency and delaying consideration of long-range goals. However, when a nurse operates with a set of clearly stated problems in mind, she can accomplish much more during the time she is working with any one patient. She may be able to work on a low priority problem at the same time she is working on a high priority one.

To say that some nursing problems will be solved and some only partly solved or delayed may seem incompatible with the concept of wholeness, yet it need not be. During the acute phase of illness or in a crisis, it is impossible for the person to focus on more than his high priority needs. To meet these needs in as thorough a manner as possible can be conducive to the wholeness of the patient. As he progresses, the way may be opened to work on other problems. In most health/illness situations the patient or family should be involved in setting priorities since they know best which problems are of greatest concern to them. They may need help in perceiving the consequences of placing a higher priority on one problem than another, and the nurse should help them examine the possibilities so that their decision can be soundly based. This involvement in determining the precedence of various aspects of care fosters personal and family integrity and a sense of responsibility. Any practice which promotes individual or family integrity is also conducive to wholeness.

Whether or not there is consensus among patient, family, and health personnel regarding the priorities set in a health/illness situation is dependent upon certain factors. Some of these factors which affect the priorities which are set include conflicting goals; external forces such as time, money, personnel; agency policy; and the value systems of the persons who are involved.

All of the nursing problems of the patient must be considered when setting priorities. The nurse should elect to deal first with those problems which have the greatest impact on his health/illness problem. In so doing, the nurse must not overlook the possibility that the side effects of nursing actions to meet one need may contribute to reaching another goal. The side effects of the involvement of a concerned, caring nurse with a patient's physical problem may go a long way toward resolving an emotional or social problem. This supports the concept of wholeness.

Another aspect of the concept of wholeness is helping the person to achieve his highest potential. Change is a slow, painful process, and helping a person reach his highest potential implies a change in the patient's behavior—in his usual patterns of functioning. He cannot cope with many changes at the same time. He can only make those changes which seem important to him. For these reasons, it is helpful to place a high priority on changes which will be of greatest significance to the patient's total welfare. It might be reiterated that the patient must be involved in deciding what those changes are.

* * * * *

It is seldom possible to attempt solutions to every nursing problem which seems desirable. Decisions must be made on which activities are important and on the rank order in which they should be arranged. There is a need in nursing to establish criteria for determining priorities. Some criteria have been established, these need to be verified and their reliability confirmed. There is a need to ascertain if criteria applied to short-term goals differ from those applied to long-term goals, and what these differences are. Criteria for setting priorities should be a part of the philosophy of any nursing service, and of any individual nurse. Some criteria which can be used to established priorities are presented below.

Criteria for Priorities for Individuals

Priorities for the individual (or the family unit) may be determined by the patient, the nurse, and/or the physician. Criteria for setting priorities include (1) preservation of life, (2) basic human needs, and (3) developmental tasks.

When the patient is able, he should be consulted regarding his own priorities. These represent what is important to him, they motivate his behavior, and they may interfere with his working to meet other needs. Should the patient's priorities seem inappropriate to the nurse, the nurse and the patient should work out this conflict and arrive at a solution that is acceptable to the patient first and to the nurse second. An example from clinical practice illustrates this point. Nurses in coronary care units are committed to performing all possible resuscitative measures to help their patients live through the cardiac crisis. A patient had been cardioverted many times, only to have a recurring life-threatening arrhythmia. It was understood by those who cared for the patient that the extent of her cardiac damage was great and the possibility of long-term survival was minimal. After experiencing another electroshock she said to the nurse, "I do not want that shock any more. I have made my peace with God and with my family. If the need arises again, please do not give me the shock." The nurse respected the patient's feelings and told her so. The nurse adjusted her priorities from those of keeping the patient alive to the patient's need for self-respect and self-determination. The patient's arrhythmia recurred; she was not cardioverted; and she died. But she died in dignity and maintained her own self-respect.

Ward rounds at the beginning of each shift provide an opportunity to find out what is high priority for the hospitalized patient. Knowing the physician's priorities for a patient can serve as a guide to the nurse in setting priorities for nursing care. For example, a physician may prescribe some treatment that confines a patient to bed, yet he requests that the person be progressively ambulated. His chief concern is that the patient be active. If the nurse is unaware of the physician's higher priority item, she may time the treatments in such a way as to markedly diminish the patient's opportunity to exercise.

Preservation of Life.

When a part of one's body must be sacrificed in order for life to continue, the life of the person takes priority over preservation of a part. This principle might be illustrated by the removal of a malignant organ or a gangrenous extremity in order to save life. While the nurse will not perform the surgery, she may help the patient see the need for it. The supportive nursing care given the patient will be toward preserving life rather than limb.

It is inevitable that priorities be determined among the various physical needs of people. Those that are necessary to the preservation of life assume more importance than comfort measures. A major discomfort such as severe pain takes precedence over a minor discomfort like temporary constipation. Most physical discomforts must be relieved to enable the person to work with other physical needs. A person in pain or other discomfort often cannot eat to meet his nutritional requirements nor sleep to meet his rest requirements until his discomforts are relieved. Although exercise is important in both therapy and rehabilitation as well as for the maintenance of health, a person who is experiencing such discomforts as pain, headache, or abdominal distention may refuse to walk until his discomfort is alleviated.

It is commonly known that air, water, and food, in that order, are essential to life. If a nurse is presented with a patient whose intravenous infusion is infiltrating, whose naso-gastric feeding tube has been dislodged, and whose tracheostomy is plugged, her knowledge of the importance of air, water, and food to human life will guide her actions as to what to do first.

Another set of guidelines for priorities in the preservation of life is indicated by the ABC's of cardiopulmonary resuscitation.[3] In a cardiac arrest, a patent airway and breathing take precedence over heart action. Not all situations in which priorities must be established among physical needs are as obvious as the above illustrations. Among physical needs, the degree of threat to life is an important criterion for deciding what to do when.

Bordicks has derived several principles that can serve as guides to action in determining priorities among physical needs.[4]

Basic Human Needs.

One useful method for determining priorities of care for an individual is derived from Maslow's hierarchy of human needs.[5] He states that physical needs come first; when these are no longer urgent, safety needs take precedence. After physical and safety needs, love needs are high in importance. When these are more or less fulfilled, needs for self-respect are paramount. And when these four areas of need are fairly well satisfied, self-actualization needs are dominant.

Little experience with people is needed to recognize the concern for physical needs which accompanies the psychological regression occurring

---

[3]James R. Jude and James O. Elam, *Fundamentals of Cardiopulmonary Resuscitation* (Philadelphia: F. A. Davis Co., 1965), pages 4-18.

[4]Katherine J. Bordicks, *Patterns of Shock*, (New York: The Macmillan Company, 1965), pages xvi-xvii.

[5]Abraham H. Maslow, *Toward a Psychology of Being* (New York: D. Van Nostrand Company, 1962), pages 19-24.

with acute illness. Matters of eating, drinking, eliminating, and relief of pain take precedence over all other needs. Efforts to explain the routines of hospital care or to prepare the patient for the expected outcomes of his illness are futile. He cannot hear what is said to him because his highest priority is focused on his physical life, on maintaining life itself. Nothing else really matters to him.

Maslow's hierarchy of human needs is of particular significance to those concerned with the rehabilitation of the handicapped. It is unlikely that a person can be motivated to reach his highest potential in spite of his disability until his physical, safety, love, and self-respect needs are fairly well gratified. The nurse whose philosophy is to help people work toward their highest potential for wholeness, a concept similar to Maslow's self-actualization, should recognize that needs first on the hierarchy must be satisfied first.

When dealing with emotional and mental illness problems, high priority is usually given to behavior which is actively destructive, outwardly toward others or to the environment or inwardly toward the self. Panic or impending panic are dealt with prior to long-standing emotional problems. In these instances, physical and safety needs are met before needs for love and self-respect.

Developmental Tasks.

Erikson's eight ages of man[6] suggest another way of determining priorities for the individual. When a person becomes ill and regresses to behavior characteristic of an earlier age level, it is quite possible that successful rehabilitation is dependent upon his progressing again through the distinctive behaviors of each age level. In other words, before a person can develop the initiative he needs to carry out a rehabilitation program, he must first learn to trust those who care for him and then he must develop a sense of autonomy. On the other hand, a geriatric patient who has not successfully dealt with the seven early stages may need a very different approach to his care than a person whose ego integrity is strong. That person may need to have some experiences provided for him so that he can learn in old age what he did not learn earlier.

The nurse who works with children and/or parents often refers to Erikson's age-related tasks. These tasks are useful criteria for setting priorities on those experiences children should have in order to develop wholesome personalities.

Criteria for Priorities Within a Group

A nurse-leader who has responsibility for several patients will have to determine priorities of care among the individuals within the group—which

[6]Erik H. Erikson, *Childhood and Society* (New York: W. W. Norton & Co., Inc., 1963), pages 247-74.

patients get minimal care, which get optimal care. Criteria for determining such priorities should be set by the agency.[7] Some criteria which help the nurse decide which patients within a group should receive a particular quality of care are discussed below.

Time.

Since the time available for nursing care is a strong determinant of priorities, it is helpful to know how much time is available. One way of estimating the amount of nursing care a patient should receive is to determine his location on a dependency scale. This scale categorizes patients according to how much they can do for themselves, from self-help to total dependency on the nurse.[8,9] For a specific category, the agency specifies a range of nursing hours per patient. With knowledge of the nursing time available for each patient, the nurse is able to make a reasonable estimate of what can be accomplished with a patient and with the total group.

Limitations of time must be considered in setting priorities. Time limits do not necessarily mean that the quality of nursing care is lessened. The intelligent use of personnel to meet the needs of the group of patients can assure quality care. This means that various nursing personnel are assigned those aspects of nursing care which they are prepared by education and experience to do well. Any other basis for assigning nurses to patients is wasteful of manpower.

When setting priorities, a decision must be made between individual and group therapy to accomplish certain goals. Nursing time can be conserved by deciding what nursing measures must be done for an individual and what can be done for a group with a similar problem. For instance, on a surgical ward several patients may need preoperative teaching. To do this for each individual may take more time than is available. All of the patients facing surgery could be assembled and one nurse could discuss with them the common elements of operative and postoperative care that all should know. This session should give opportunity for questions, for sharing of ideas and concerns. Another solution could be that a videotape be prepared by the nursing staff, and the tape played for viewing by the patients. Then a nurse could lead a discussion of the material presented on the videotape. This could further conserve nursing time. Granted, these may not be ideal ways of meeting patient's needs for preoperative teaching, but it is better than no teaching program. For those patients who may

---

[7]Ruth B. Freeman, *Public Health Nursing Practice* (Philadelphia: W. B. Saunders Company, 1963), pages 273-5.

[8]John P. Young, *A Method for Allocation of Nursing Personnel to Meet Impatient Care Needs* (Baltimore: Johns Hopkins Hospital Operations Research Division, 1962).

[9]Lauraine A. Thomas, Chairman, Task Force IV, *Establishing Staffing Patterns Based on Acuity of Patient Needs* (San Francisco: California Nurses' Association, November, 1968).

need additional instruction, it could be given before or after the group session.

In arriving at one or the other of these solutions, one must not overlook the support that comes to the individual patient in belonging to a group, in seeing that he is not alone. When available nursing time is at a premium, the high priority for individual instruction may have to give way for the lower priority group method. However, whenever group methods of dealing with problems are a choice, it is important to look at both the advantages and disadvantages of the individual *versus* group methods so that proper priority can be given to each. The serendipities of group therapy may outweigh the advantages of one-to-one therapy.

Vulnerability.

In addition to time, vulnerability is another high-priority criterion. The more vulnerable the patient, the higher his priority within a group. Vulnerability refers to the patient's susceptibility to disease, trauma, relapse, death, or other personal threat. He is defenseless. He cannot meet his own needs. The very young and the very old are usually more vulnerable than those in between. The more helpless a person is—physically, mentally, or emotionally helpless—the more vulnerable he is. It is usually true that the higher a person is on the dependency scale, the more vulnerable he is. The critically ill or injured are highly vulnerable. These patients are placed high on priority for care, a significant reason for intensive and coronary care units.

Prognosis.

In contrast to vulnerability as a criterion is prognosis. If the person is returned to health, will his life expectancy and his contribution to society be proportional to the needs the group must forego so that the individual's needs can be met, Prenatal patients, children, and persons with communicable diseases often are given a higher priority than geriatric patients with long-term illnesses. Among the problems of emotional or mental illness, aggression and depression receive attention prior to paranoid or sociopathic tendencies. Current philosophy of many community health facilities places a higher priority on crisis intervention than on long-term care. Their rationale is the greatest good for the most people or the best good for those who can contribute most to society.

Normal versus Disaster Situation.

Priorities for the care of individuals in a group differ in normal and in disaster situations.[10] Disaster triage places highest priority on the person

[10]Robert F. Mahoney, *Emergency and Disaster Nursing* (New York: The Macmillan Company, 1967), pages 50-52.

who has the greatest possibility of quick return to the community with minimal care. The lowest priority is given the most critically ill or injured who have the lowest probability of survival. This is different from what occurs on the typical hospital service. Whether there should be this difference between disaster and normal care is debatable. Ethical and moral questions are posed by the high costs of medical and nursing care for meeting the needs of the critically ill in preference to meeting the needs of the less ill. Is it morally right to focus so much care on one person and perhaps deprive many of a more abundant life? Consider the time, equipment, effort, and skilled personnel needed to treat the acute phases of the high incidence diseases in society: heart disease, cerebrovascular accidents, chronic lung disease. In normal times, should a higher priority be placed on prevention than on treatment of these conditions?

To determine the priorities of individuals within groups, not only the time, vulnerability, and prognosis of the individual and normalcy of the situation must be considered, but also the ethical and moral questions must be asked—and answered.

Criteria For Priorities of Nursing Services

In general, the content of this book focuses on planning patient care for individuals and for small groups of patients. However, to do this the nurse must also consider the demands of the community for nursing services. Whether working with individual or community health problems, the process is similar. Some guidelines for setting priorities for nursing services within a community have been established by Freeman.[11] In selecting priorities for nursing services within a community, it is essential that professional nurses participate in the decisions, in establishing policies, and in implementing new services or phasing out unneeded services.

* * * * *

Assessment is the first step of the nursing process and is essential for the planning of individualized patient care. Assessment consists of the collection of data about the patient from a variety of sources and the categorization of these data into problem areas. The data are categorized for the purpose of identifying nursing problems presented by the patient. Once nursing problems are identified and priorities are set, the second step of the nursing process, intervention, begins.

---

[11] Freeman, *op. cit.*

REFERENCES

*Abdellah, Faye G. "Methods of Identifying Covert Aspects of Nursing Problems." *Nursing Research* 6:1(1957):4-23.

Abdellah, Faye, *et. al. Patient-Centered Approaches to Nursing.* New York: The Macmillan Company, 1960.

*Bonney, Virginia, and Rothberg, June. *Nursing Diagnosis and Therapy.* New York: National League for Nursing, 1963.

Bordicks, Katherine J. *Patterns of Shock.* New York: The Macmillan Company, 1965.

*Chambers, Wilda. "Nursing Diagnosis." *American Journal of Nursing* 62:11 (1962):102-4.

*Durand, Mary, and Prince, Rosemary, "Nursing Diagnosis: Process and Decision." *Nursing Forum* V:4(1966):50-63.

Erickson, Erik H. *Childhood and Society.* New York: W. W. Norton & Company, Inc., 1963.

Freeman, Ruth B. *Public Health Nursing Practice.* Philadelphia: W. B. Saunders Company, 1963.

Henderson, Virginia. *Basic Principles of Nursing Care.* London: International Council of Nurses, 1961.

*Juntti, M. Jeanette. "Problem Solving in Arranging for Comprehensive Home Care. *Nursing Forum* VIII:1(1969):103-9.

Komorita, Nori I. "Nursing Diagnosis." *American Journal of Nursing* 63:12 (1963):83-6.

Mahoney, Robert F. *Emergency and Disaster Nursing.* New York: The Macmillan Company, 1967.

Maslow, Abraham H. *Toward a Psychology of Being.* New York: D. Van Nostrand Company, 1962.

Moore, Larry. "Problem Recognition in Nursing Service Administration." *Nursing Forum* VIII:1(1969):94-102.

*Nite, Gladys, and Willis, Frank. *The Coronary Patient.* New York: The Macmillan Company, 1964.

Venger, Mary Jane. "Hyperbaric Oxygenation: Nursing Responsibility in Planning for a New Clinical Service." *Nursing Clinics of North America* 1:1(1966):131-42.

Yura, Helen, and Walsh, Mary B. *The Nursing Process.* Washington. D. C.; Catholic University Press, 1967.

CLINICAL EXPERIENCE

1. Using three different nursing histories (Assignment #1, Chapter III) and other assessment data from the patients, categorize the data into problem areas. Identify the problems or needs of the patients. Compare the types of problems identified with the method of taking a nursing history.
2. Set priorities on the problems identified for one person. Defend your selection of top priority problem.
3. Consider the nursing needs of the patients assigned to one nurse team leader. Decide which patient(s) should have high priority for optimal nursing care. What common needs of several patients could be met by group therapy?
4. Investigate one community health problem and find out what nurses are doing to help solve the problem. What criteria were used to establish the priority of the problem?

---

*Suggested for additional reading.

Chapter 5

Intervention—Planning

Three major steps—assessment, intervention, and evaluation—constitute the nursing process. Each step influences and is influenced by the others. The intervention step of the nursing process is what the nurse does to help the person solve his nursing problems or to meet his needs. Intervention is the planning, doing phase of nursing. It must follow a careful assessment; it cannot be done in an effective way without this. Inadequate planning may result in uncoordinated or purposeless nursing actions. Unless intervention is followed by evaluation, there is no way of knowing whether the action taken met the person's needs.

Part of nursing intervention may or may not be in the patient's presence. This is the planning of ways by which nursing can help the person with his problems. Another part of intervention consists of what the nurse does for and with the person in a one-to-one relationship during which the nurse ministers to the needs of the patient, listens to and converses with him, and teaches or counsels him. It might be said that there is a thinking-planning phase of nursing intervention and a doing-interacting phase. Both planning and acting are essential components of nursing intervention. Both may involve various types of nursing personnel.

The act of planning is a complex one. It is a thinking, decision-making process. The planning of nursing care consists of the formulation of objectives, devising alternative ways of achieving objectives, selecting approaches, and deciding who does what and when. The foundation on which planning is built is knowledge and judgment. The purpose of the planning is to develop a set of nursing actions which will help the person with his health/illness problems. The set of nursing actions which are written down as a reference for all nurses caring for the patient is called the nursing care plan.

ELEMENTS OF PLANNING

What is Planning ?

Serving as a guide for the solution of problems and the attainment of objectives, planning is an important part of professional nursing practice because it presents an orderly pattern of nursing care designed to meet the patient's needs.

Planning is decision-making. Decisions must be made regarding the objectives for patient care. The objectives should not only help solve the patient's problem but must be feasible within the agency and must harmonize with the philosophy of nursing held by the nurse and the agency. There may be more than one objective for some nursing problems. In that event, the objectives of nursing care must be ranked according to priority. It may be necessary to decide whether some objectives may safely be omitted from the plan.

Decisions must be made as to which of several alternative approaches are used and in what order. When writing nursing orders, the nurse decides on the timing and sequence of care, the kind of nurse best able to give each type of care, and the adaptations of care required by the patient.

Decisions! *Decisions!* DECISIONS! They are the stuff of which planning is made. The making of a decision entails weighing the evidence and taking a risk. The risk is minimized by a thorough knowledge of the patient, by careful analysis of the problem, and by sound clinical judgment based on education and experience.

Planning is more than decision-making. It includes the creation of a pattern or design for action and the implementation of the design.

Why is Planning Necessary?

A plan helps to organize and give direction, guidance, and meaning to what is done for and with the person needing nursing service. Without a plan, service is haphazard and aimless. A plan saves time and energy by minimizing repetition of instructions and by providing essential information about the patient's nursing care to each person who gives care.

Since a patient's condition is seldom static, his needs for nursing care vary from time to time. To keep up with these changing needs, the nursing care plan must be up-dated with each change in need. Planning then becomes a continuous process and a written plan of care is the best way of informing the staff of the modifications of the patient's nursing care.

In many agencies nursing is a twenty-four-hour-a-day, seven-day-a-week service, so there must be some way of coordinating the efforts of nursing personnel toward a common goal. Without a plan to which all nursing personnel can refer, there can be no assurance of a goal-directed service to patients. Without a plan, nurses on various shifts and on different days cannot work in harmony to meet the needs of patients. A plan can help to synchronize and organize the actions of all nursing staff for the best interests of the patient. As nursing personnel share information and observations about the patient, the plan can be developed, revised, and updated to adjust to new knowledge and to the changing condition of the patient. A plan is a medium of communication among all the nursing personnel involved in the care of the patient.

Even in agencies in which only one nurse is involved with a patient, a plan is necessary. The plan outlines the goals, approaches, and expected outcomes of the nursing intervention. It guides the nurse in her care and assures continuity of care should another nurse be assigned to the patient.

If nursing is indeed a profession, it must offer to people a service which contributes to their welfare. Professions are distinguished by their dedication to the achievement of objectives for those they serve. Professional nurses then must be able to formulate objectives for their service and must have some orderly means of achieving those objectives. This is what planning is all about. For the solution of most problems or the attainment of objectives, a nursing care plan would seem to be an important part of professional nursing practice.

Who Does the Planning?

Planning may be done by an individual nurse, by a nurse in consultation with selected resource people, by the nursing team, or by some combination of these. In any case, the data concerning the patient and the problems previously identified are available for the planning of the care. Solutions to common problems may be devised by the nurse team leader. Likewise, adapting routine care to the patient's desires and habitual patterns can usually be done most efficiently by the team leader. In the interest of saving time, it is wise for the team leader alone to write the nursing orders for common nursing problems and for adapting general care to the patient's desires.

For the solution of high priority, difficult, or perplexing problems, the nurse may confer with consultants or with other members of the health team, such as physicians and physical therapists. The ideas of a group can be creative and varied in devising approaches to problems and in determining ways of applying new concepts and theories. The patient and/or family may participate in the planning.

Even though there is sharing in the planning process, the nurse team leader, the nurse ultimately responsible for the patient's care, is the one who composes the nursing care plan. In general, the better prepared by education and experience the nurse is, the more complete, objective, and successful will be the nursing care plan she develops.

How is Planning Done?

Before any planning can be done, a certain amount of knowledge is essential. All of the information about the patient acquired in the assessment step should be available for use in planning. Some of the assessment data will be used to adapt nursing measures to the desires of the patient. Very little planning is needed before writing these adaptations of care into the nursing care plan. Timing and sequence of care, food and fluid preferences, rest and sleep routines may not need any deliberative process to determine what to include in the nursing care plan. The largest part of planning time should be devoted to developing solutions to problems.

For many of the common problems presented by the patient, the educational and experiential background of the nursing team will provide enough resources to design the nursing care. Yet it is highly probable that one or more of the problems presented by the patient are unusual enough to demand the use of other resources to identify the nursing care needed.

Those who plan nursing care should have time to do library research on nursing problems and time to consult more experienced persons in order to devise adequate nursing care plans. The nurse-team leader need not be the only one who seeks out this information. The staff nurse directly involved in the care of the patient may be the one who does the library research. Without the opportunity to study both the common and the unusual problems, nurses cannot grow and develop. Nursing approaches soon become stereotyped and hackneyed, and the gap between theory and practice widens. Therefore, a determined effort must be made in every agency where nursing is practiced to provide resources and to require nursing personnel to use them. All members of the nursing team must have access to and read current nursing literature. Knowledge of current literature will give the nurse innovative as well as conventional ways of meeting nursing needs of people.

Innovation and creativity in the solution of nursing problems are more often the by-product of a search for knowledge than of a task-oriented approach to nursing. Designing experimental solutions to nursing problems requires time, energy, and the use of resources. Experimentation and innovation are vital to the progress of nursing and must be carried out by the progressive practitioner. It cannot all be left to the researcher or the graduate student. For some people, day-dreaming and "think-time" are productive of creative and innovative ideas. For others, exhaustive library work with a deliberate effort to apply principles and ideas to the practice of nursing may result in new ways of attacking nursing problems. One way to extract nursing implications from non-nursing literature is to read widely on one problem area and, while reading, continually ask, "What does this tell me about ways to assess the patient in order to identify his problem?

What nursing intervention is suggested by the way others have attacked this problem? What evaluation criteria have others used which can be adapted to nursing?

An attempt to summarize the areas in which the nurse may need to increase her knowledge relative to patient's problems seems futile. Some of the more obvious areas involve new treatments and medications, the meaning of behavior, ways to alter signs and symptoms, unusual medical diagnoses, the culture or ethnic background of the patient, the types of community services available for an extraordinary problem.

Initiation of planning occurs with recognition of problems and with the need to personalize the care of the patient. Equipped with assessment data, the identified problems and the knowledge necessary to utilize the information, the nurse proceeds with planning. The team leader initiates the planning session by presenting the data from the patient and the problems which were identified. The leader or a designated team member may then present her findings from library research or consultation. With this preface, discussion begins with formulating the nursing objectives which seem appropriate and ranking these in order of priority. The group then suggests alternative courses of action which might achieve the objectives and the most desirable approaches to try first. The leader will guide the discussion, will encourage participation of all members of the team, and will summarize the content of the discussion at the close of the session. A team member may be assigned to record the suggestions of the group during the session. The leader will write on the nursing care plan the problem, objectives, and proposed actions. In addition to the items concerning problems, the team leader will use assessment data to write other nursing orders to personalize the care of the patient—ways in which care is adapted to the patient's desires. The team leader should also record the outcomes of the planning conference on the patient's permanent record, listing alternatives that may be tried if those selected fail to meet the objectives. The film, "Mrs. Reynolds Needs a Nurse"[1] graphically portrays a team conference in which problems are identified and a variety of approaches are suggested.

For some problems the patient or family should be involved in the planning. They may help formulate objectives, set priorities, design and select alternative approaches for meeting their needs. When their wishes regarding care are consulted, the care will be more acceptable to them and the probability of success of the plan greatly enhanced. Especially should the patient or family be involved in planning concerned with rehabilitation and promotion of healthful living.

[1]Available from the A.N.A.-N.L.N. film library.

FORMULATING OBJECTIVES

Objectives are statements of the changes in behavior of the patient which will be brought about by nursing actions. These changes in behavior should signify that the patient's health/illness problems have been solved insofar as nursing can contribute to the solution. Nursing objectives describe the intended outcome of the nursing action. They show what the practice of nursing can contribute to the solution of health/illness problems. These objectives are written on the nursing care plan. Space should be provided on the form used for nursing care plans to list nursing objectives and the nursing actions designed to achieve those objectives.

While formulating objectives for the nursing care of a patient, the nurse must consider both his immediate and his future needs. Short-term goals have to do with immediate needs arising from the present status of the patient, his stage of dependency, his symptoms. Long-range objectives pertain to nursing measures related to rehabilitation needs, the prevention of complications and exacerbations of disease or additional illness. Other long-range goals pertain to teaching the patient or family what they need to know for self-care or more healthful living, helping the patient achieve his highest potential for wholeness, or controlling the disease in the community.

At the outset of planning the nursing care of a patient it is essential that both short-term and long-range goals be envisioned. The achievement of long-range goals may indicate immediate nursing measures. One prime example is the goal that a bed-ridden patient will have no pressure sores. Unless preventive measures are initiated while the skin is still in good condition, what is done may be futile and prevention will be replaced by therapy. Prevention of disease by immunization or by healthful living is a long-range goal. Unless the need for prevention is anticipated early in the care of the patient and procedures are begun before actual risk of a disease occurs, the effectiveness of the program is limited.

When planning nursing care, it is important to formulate as many objectives as are indicated by the patient's problems. While working with a patient the nurse often may contribute to the achievement of several objectives as easily as she might work toward one objective. She may miss the opportunity if she is unaware of the various objectives formulated for the patient. For instance, while helping a person with some physical activity, such as eating or walking, the conversation may be guided into a topic concerned with a teaching or counseling objective.

Behavioral Objectives

Some helpful guidelines for formulating objectives can be gleaned from Mager's book on preparing objectives.[2] If one applies his concept of an

[2]Robert Mager, *Preparing Instructional Objectives* (Palo Alto: Fearon Publishers, Inc., 1962).

instructional objective to a nursing objective, she can describe a meaningfully stated nursing objective as one which communicates to the staff the intent of the nurse(s) who stated it. Mager declared that the objective must describe what the learner will be doing as a result of what he has learned. "The statement which communicates best will be one which describes the terminal behavior of the learner well enough to preclude misinterpretation."[3] A well-stated nursing objective should state what the patient will be able to do as a result of nursing care. The objective should describe the patient's behavior change so well that all who care for the patient will have the same picture. *Behavior* in this instance is broadly used to signify physiologic, psychosocial, or intellectual behavior as well as activities of daily living.

In contrast to behaviorally stated objectives are objectives which state what the nurse will do for the patient. These objectives are stated as "to accept . . .," "to promote . . .," "to prevent . . .," "to maintain . . .," "to prepare . . . " This type of objective infers that nursing is doing something *to* a patient rather than that nursing is a service aimed at changing the outcomes of the patient's health/illness problems by working *with* him, by increasing his own capabilities. An example of a behaviorally stated nursing objective might be: "able to take care of own colostomy." An objective stating what the nurse will do for the patient is: "to teach colostomy care." The first example is more measurable than the second. The first is more likely to show that nursing made a difference in the outcome of the patient's problem. Stating objectives in terms of the change in patient behavior suggests the nurse must specify what the patient will be doing or what behavior will be evidenced when he "accepts" his diagnosis or bed-rest or change in role. These objectives will indicate the terminal behavior when a patient has been "prepared" for surgery, when healing has been "promoted," when respiratory complications have been "prevented," when a patent airway is "provided," when adequate nutrition is "maintained," or when a therapeutic environment is "created."

To specify terminal behavior of patients as a result of nursing actions requires that the nurse be able to predict the outcomes of her actions. To predict with a fair degree of accuracy, the nurse must weigh the evidence about the patient in its proper perspective. She must have the knowledge applicable to the situation. She must have the discernment to use that knowledge in an unbiased manner.

Evaluation Criteria

Terminal behavior which is the outcome of nursing objectives can be considered as evaluation criteria. These criteria, identified during the planning phase of the nursing process, are essential to the evaluation step of the nursing process. Data from the patient relative to these criteria will provide

---

[3]Mager, *Preparing Instructional Objectives,* p. 11

evidence that the nursing care was successful or unsuccessful in reaching goals. As defined by Mager,[4] evaluation criteria should be measurable, observable, describable in unambiguous terms, so that all those concerned with evaluating the objective know what to expect and will recognize behavior change when it occurs.

The precise description of evaluation criteria is crucial to the development of the science of nursing. Because of the nature of nursing and the stage of development of nursing science, the criteria now used to evaluate nursing are more subjective and less precise than is desirable. Often, there is difficulty in identifying the specific changes produced by nursing. It is not known as yet how to describe some of the specific changes in patient behavior resulting from nursing care. Neither are nurses very proficient in describing nursing actions in specific, exact terms so that those actions can be duplicated by another nurse. But, until they try—consistently, continuously, and thoughtfully as individuals within a developing profession—nurses cannot derive this knowledge. As the science of nursing improves, more precise criteria for measuring the effects of nursing will be developed. The effort must be made, and attempts of each nurse must be shared, compared, and contrasted with those of other nurses if a nursing science is to be derived. Researchers and practitioners should be committed to discovering and perfecting objective measures of the effectiveness of nursing care.

Evaluation criteria may include anything about the person which can be noticed by another person. Measures may be physiological data, such as a change in heart rate or rhythm, blood pressure, temperature or urine output. Emotional or psychological measures may include the amount and type of social interaction, the presence or absence of crying, withdrawal, denial, or hostility. Evaluation may be based on what the patient says or how well he performs some act. Verbalization about relief of a subjective symptom, enjoyment of food, change of mood or attitude, whether or not he follows through on a referral, are all data that can indicate that an objective has been reached.

Laboratory and X-ray examinations may be accepted as evidence that certain nursing objectives have been reached. A negative chest X-ray might indicate that a deep-breathing, coughing, turning program was effective in preventing atelectasis. A normal blood or urine sugar would indicate that a diabetic probably is following his dietary and exercise program. An electrocardiogram might serve as evidence that the rest program and environmental control for a cardiac patient was improving his cardiac status. Simple tests for urine sugar or acetone, blood in excretions, pH or specific gravity of body fluids provide measurable data about the patient's physiologic behavior. Nurses have available many accurate tools which

---

[4]Mager, *Preparing Instructional Objectives,* p. 43.

can and should be used to evaluate nursing care. Examples of some common measuring devices are tape measures for measuring circumference of edematous parts, protractor-type goniometers for measuring range of joint motion. Scales, thermometers, and spirometers also provide objective measures.

Because of man's wholeness, the interrelationships of parts to whole, physiologic measures may sometimes be used to evaluate emotional, social, or spiritual behavior change. When measurement of emotional and social behavior changes cannot be done with mechanical devices, behavioral change can be described in objective terms and terminology can be used which is commonly understood by all concerned with evaluating care.

During the planning of care, a team conference is helpful not only for prescribing nursing actions but for arriving at a consensus on the terminal behavior expected of the patient as a result of the nursing actions. Descriptions of terminal behavior should be discussed until all personnel have a clear picture of the desired outcomes of nursing intervention.

Conditional Outcomes

Sometimes it may be necessary to include in the statement of the objective certain restrictions or constraints which are imposed on the patient as he performs the intended act. These restrictions may specify the conditions under which the patient will perform the desired action or will describe the people, appliances, or therapeutic factors which may aid him in performing the action. Some examples of objectives which describe terminal behavior and specify a restriction follow:

> Mr. J. will be able to walk alone with a cane a distance of ten yards and ascend and descend three steps.

The restrictions imposed on Mr. J. are the cane and his aloneness. The terminal act, or evaluation criterion, is his ability to walk the specified distance and get up and down three steps.

> Given a menu from a restaurant, Mr. K. will select a meal within his calorie and sodium restrictions.

The condition in this objective is the menu from a restaurant. The terminal act, or criterion for evaluation, is that the food selected will be appropriate to his dietary prescription.

> Without assistance, Mrs. L. will be able to get out of bed by transferring to a wheelchair placed parallel to the right side of her bed.

The restriction on Mrs. L. is that she have no assistance. She will be able to transfer herself from bed to wheelchair as a result of nursing actions.

Time is one constraint that nursing might consider placing on nursing objectives. With rising costs of medical and nursing care, every effort must be made to accomplish the most in the least amount of time. Time limits might be imposed on the achievements of patients. These limits, of course, should be reasonable and within what is usually considered a normal time span for achieving the desired goal. Setting such limits might require some daring on the part of nurses, but it also can furnish incentive and motivation to reach these goals. Some examples of objectives in which time limits are imposed follow.

> By her fourth postoperative day, Mrs. N. will be able to take care of her own personal hygiene needs.
>
> By his seventh postoperative day, Mr. O. will be able to assemble materials and do his own colostomy irrigation.
>
> Within ten days of his C.V.A., Mr. P. will be able to feed himself, turn himself in bed, and sit on the side of the bed without help.
>
> After three home visits, Miss O. will be able to give her own insulin after correctly testing and interpreting her urine sugar analysis.

The time limits should not be so rigid that individual differences or extenuating circumstances are not taken into consideration.

Practical Considerations

To write as many behaviorally stated nursing objectives as the care of one patient might involve and to do this for all the patients with whom a nurse works is a formidable task. It is time-consuming, thought-provoking, and precision-oriented. It is an educational experience and is valuable in both nursing education and nursing practice. It demands the application of all the knowledge a nurse has. It requires clear, precise thinking, specificity, and conceptual ability. It is intellectually stimulating and promotes professional growth. It gives goal-direction to the work of the nurse and, when she sees the results of her efforts by measurable criteria, her job satisfaction and her sense of personal worth may be enhanced.

Still, one must be practical. Planning must not be such a complicated process that the patient is deprived of the direct care a nurse can give. There are some ways of increasing the practicability of writing nursing objectives and listing evaluation criteria. Grouping together patients with similar problems means that similar objectives and evaluation criteria may apply to several patients. Sometimes, one nursing objective might contribute to more than one nursing problem. When this can be done, nursing time is conserved and more is accomplished in the time available. When a nurse first starts to write behaviorally stated nursing objectives, the process is difficult and time-consuming. With continued practice in writing objectives and growth in clinical experience, the process becomes easier and quicker.

For hospitalized patients, certain types of general care are common to many patients. These include personal hygiene measures, attention to eating, drinking, elimination, recording vital signs, intake and output. So long as the nurse adapts this care to the individual patient and there is no major clinical or long-term problem associated with these measures, it is not necessary to write detailed objectives on them. Her experience and education should have equipped the nurse to perform these measures safely, to personalize them to the patient, and to evaluate care constructively. This shortcut could leave more time for perfecting the objectives and evaluation criteria for major, high-priority or long-term problems.

Inservice educational programs might focus a few sessions on writing objectives and on specifying evaluation criteria to improve the skill of the practitioner. A card file or pocket-size notebook might be compiled which classifies nursing objectives and criteria for evaluating the degree of attainment of objectives. Additions to the list could be made from time to time. By referring to the card file or notebook, the time spent in planning care could be shortened.

Emphasis can be placed on the formulation of objectives with appropriate evaluation criteria in the education of students of nursing. During the course of their nursing education, students should become quite skilled in writing objectives. One way in which nursing education might improve clinical practice in the agencies used for clinical experience is to have the students share with the staff the nursing objectives and evaluation criteria they outline for patients. Together, students and staff might work on a compilation of nursing objectives and evaluation criteria which could serve as a handy reference for nurses who plan patient care.

Some nurses may elect to state certain objectives in greater detail than others. Probably the nurse will place a high priority on fully developing those objectives derived from a few health/illness problems with which she is primarily concerned. For instance, a nurse in a coronary care unit might compile objectives concerned with improving heart action or circulation and with the acceptance of bed-rest. A nurse dealing with many cancer patients might have detailed objectives dealing with pain and acceptance of terminal illness. A community health nurse in an economically deprived area might concentrate on objectives for improving nutrition or for utilizing available community services. A nurse in a rehabilitation center would be primarily concerned with patients being able to perform the activities of daily living. The suggestion that nurses focus their attention on fully developing a few selected objectives is made because of the limitations of time and personnel with which most nurses work. All health/illness problems must be considered, but some may be handled in a more cursory manner. In any event, the nursing objective and evaluation criteria must be personalized to the patient. The same goal may be evaluated in different ways for different patients.

* * * *

In summary, a well-stated nursing objective will give evidence of one or more of these characteristics:

1. It will specify in exact terms the behavior of the patient which is the expected outcome of nursing care.
2. It will describe any conditions imposed on the patient in the performance of the expected behavior.
3. It will describe how well the patient will be able to perform the behavior to be considered acceptable.

Following are some examples of problems, objectives, and evaluation criteria.

Problem: Unable to sleep.
Objective: Without the aid of medication, Mrs. B. will be able to sleep at least six hours every night.
Evaluation criterion: number of hours slept.

Problem: Pain and inflammation at site of I.V. puncture.
Objective: Mr. C. will show no signs of inflammation and will say there is no pain at site of I.V.
Evaluation criteria: no signs of inflammation at I.V. site; no pain, swelling, heat, redness. Mr. C. states he has no pain there.

Problem: Constipation with straining.
Objective: Mrs. D. will have a soft stool every 1-2 days without straining.
Evaluation criteria: soft stool, bowels move every 1-2 days, no straining.

Problem: Poor circulation to feet.
Objective: Mr. E. will have warm, pink feet with intact skin and subcutaneous tissue.
Evaluation criteria: feet warm to touch, pink color, Mr. E. says feet are warm, no skin lesions, no discoloration of skin, no subcutaneous lumps, rapid capillary refilling time.

Problem: Unable to accept therapeutic diet.
Objective: Mrs. F. will express satisfaction with meals and will eat at least ¾ of the food on each tray.
Evaluation criteria: expressions of satisfaction with food, amount of food eaten. (Weight change could be a criterion.)

Problem: Needs to understand therapeutic diet.
Objective #1: Mrs. F. will be able to write out menus for each meal for a week.
Evaluation criteria: week's menus o.k.'d by dietitian as appropriate to diet.
Objective #2: Given a menu from a restaurant, Mrs. F. will be able to select a meal consistent with diet.
Evaluation criteria: marks menu and identifies quantities appropriate to diet.

Problem: Unable to return to usual occupation.
Objective: Mr. G. will have a plan for work by the time he is dismissed from the hospital.
Evaluation criteria: has a plan acceptable to him, can describe it, and knows where to get employment or training needed.

Problem: Dyspnea.
Objective: Mr. H. will be able to breathe without effort when lying at an angle of less than 20 degrees.
Evaluation criteria: breathes without effort, does not use accessory muscles of respiration when lying at less than 20°.

SELECTING ALTERNATIVES

Planning the care of a patient is a multi-faceted process. Once objectives for the care have been formulated, the next step is to contrive various nursing approaches which might help achieve the goals. Approaches, as used here, refer to the nursing activities clustered around a nursing objective—what nursing can do toward achieving the objective. The nature of these approaches will be discussed in Chapter 6. This section deals with methods of selecting from several proposed approaches those which will be used.

Ideally, the selection of alternative approaches should be done by a nursing team in a team conference. When several people contribute ideas, more diversified approaches may be devised. The patient himself may be included in the conference. The patient or family can offer impressive guidance in the selection of alternative approaches to problems. Their awareness of what is or is not acceptable to the patient and/or family is knowledge the nurse may not have, yet it is vital to selection of a desirable approach. Other sources might aid in designing or selecting alternative approaches. Assessment data provide important clues regarding what is acceptable to the patient. Textbooks, other references, and past experience are helpful resources for possible approaches as well as for indicating the probability that the action will achieve the desired result. In practice, past experience is one of the most useful resources for these decisions.

Once a number of approaches have been outlined, the nurse or nursing team must select those which may be feasible and those which should be rejected. The proposed nursing actions become hypotheses to test to see if they do indeed contribute to the solution of the problem. Which hypothesis is selected for initial testing is based on a consideration of the probability of success in reaching the goal and the desirability of its effects. For instance, for objective *A*, three different approaches are proposed. It might be hypothesized that approach *X* will achieve objective *A*, that approach *Y* will achieve objective *A* and that approach Z will not achieve objective *A*. Approach Z is then rejected. Selection between approach *X* and approach *Y* is based on critical thinking regarding the possible results or consequences of the proposed nursing action. What are all the possible effects of doing or not doing the proposed action? What is the probability that the proposed action will produce one result or another? How valuable, how desirable is the result of the proposed nursing action? Will this result be a significant or an insignificant factor in reaching the goal? That hypothesis selected first, has a high probability of achieving the desired results and a high value in terms of effectiveness.

Sometimes compromises must be made. One alternative may have a very high probability of achieving a result, but the result may be more temporary or not so important or less acceptable to the patient than some other alternative whose probability is lower. One approach may have side effects which preclude its usage. If the proposed approach seemed to be a very effective method of achieving the objective, yet was undesirable to some other member of the health team, another approach may need to be selected. In some instances, the desirability of an approach to other team members, as well as to the patient, must be considered. In either case, the choice of action may be the one with a lower probability and a higher desirability. If the planning group is unable to decide on the merits of approach *X* over approach *Y*, it might be hypothesized that the probability of approach *X* for achieving objective *A* is greater than approach *Y*. In this instance, both approaches may need to be tested and objectively evaluated to see which is the more desirable.

In order to facilitate the choice of an approach, the degree of probability and desirability that the consequences of the action will achieve the objective may be indicated on a scale of numerical or symbolic values.[5] At this time in the development of nursing as a profession, exact numerical values cannot be stated in a given situation. If and when such a system is developed, the computer will be a tremendous aid in this phase of planning patient care. However, in the present stage of development, a scale of estimated values would be useful as a tool of communication among those concerned with the nursing care of the patient. The scale could contain from three to five, perhaps ten, gradations to indicate levels of probability and desirability. The important feature must be that the scale communicates the idea to those who use the system so that the numbers or symbols have similar meaning to all who use them. An example of a scale is given below.

To illustrate the foregoing discussion, a clinical example concerning the problem of postoperative pain is given.

> Mrs. J. is a 42-year-old mother of four children. She is five feet four inches tall, weighing 165 lbs. This is her third day after a cholecystectomy. She is complaining of moderate incisional pain, has some abdomi-

[5]Frederick J. McDonald and Mary T. Harms, "Theoretical Model for an Experimental Curriculum," *Nursing Outlook* 14:8(1966):48-51.

nal distention and occasionally passes flatus. She is restless and irritable and has a low tolerance for pain. Respirations are shallow. She has P.R.N. orders for meperidine HCl. (Demerol) 50 mg. (I.M.) or propoxyphene HCl. (Darvon) 65 mg. The nursing objective is: Mrs. J's pain will be relieved enough to permit rest and relaxation. Evaluation criteria are: Mrs. J's hand, face, and neck muscles are relaxed, Mrs. J. says she is comfortable, lies quietly in bed, says pain is minimal.

Approach *X* might be to give Mrs. J. the Demerol. The consequences of this action would be (1) quick relief of pain, which is both highly probable and highly desirable, and (2) possible depression of gastro-intestinal motility and of respiration, causing more discomfort from distention and possible lung complications. This consequence is moderately probable and highly undesirable. Approach *Y* would be to give Mrs. J. the Darvon, and, as soon as it diminishes her pain to assist her to walk, after which she would be returned to bed, positioned so as to enhance release of flatus and minimize tension on her incision. The possible results of this approach would be (1) moderate probability of relief of pain which is highly desirable, and (2) minimal adverse effect of drug with good possibility of relieving distention and promoting respiration. These consequences would be moderately probable and highly desirable. Approach Z might be to position Mrs. J. so as to promote passage of flatus and tell her that this will relieve her pain. This approach might be rejected because Mrs. J's low tolerance for pain would preclude the possibility of this action being effective. As shown in the Table 5.1, the selection of Approach *Y* would be made because its score for probability and desirability is higher than that of approach *X*.

Table 5.1
Selection of Alternatives for Objective *A*

	Consequence	*Probability*	*Desirability*	*Score*
Approach *X*	1	+++	+++	
	2	++	0	8+
Approach *Y*	1	++	+++	
	2	++	+++	10+
Approach Z		0	+	1+

Code: High= +++
Moderate= ++
Low= +
Unlikely= 0

Under some circumstances the selection of alternatives is not an either/or decision but is concerned with the order or sequence in which various approaches are tried. For instance, when a nurse sees a dyspneic patient, she might consider doing all of these things: pull the patient up in bed, turn on oxygen, give a P.R.N. medication, or sit by the bed and hold the patient's hand while trying to find out if an emotional problem is contributing to the dyspnea. For a particular patient, all of the approaches may be desirable and have a good probability of success. Which is done first would be based on knowledge of the total situation. What is important is that the nurse could quickly recognize the problem, see the alternatives, and have the prior knowledge necessary to decide the sequence in which she should try the various approaches.

There is a danger on a busy service, though, that alternatives are not thought through nor given due consideration. Many nurses, when dealing with the common problem of pain, simply give the prescribed medication without considering an alternative course of action. This is strikingly portrayed in a study reported by Mary B. Tarasuk, Julina Rhymes, and Robert Leonard. Patients complaining of pain were divided into two groups. Those in the experimental group were given the opportunity to discuss their discomfort with the nurse. Patients in the control group were given pain medication when they complained of pain; there was little, if any, communication between nurse and patient. In the experimental group, the alternative of giving pain medication was selected 31 percent of the time as compared with 100 percent for the control group. For the remaining 69 percent of the experimental group, alternative comfort measures were selected to relieve the pain. The relief of pain was more marked and quicker in the experimental group than in the control group.[6] From time to time every nurse should honestly ask herself if she is considering alternative approaches to common, everyday problems.

To develop creative and innovative approaches to any nursing problem requires the deliberative, critical thinking outlined above. Each practitioner should have the time, energy, and desire to develop creative and innovative approaches to nursing problems from time to time. Hopefully this will not be relegated only to the student, the researcher, or the clinical specialist. Rather, each nurse will come to know the joy and stimulation which can come from such an activity. It should be both a criterion for and a symbol of professional excellence.

THE NURSING CARE PLAN

Culmination of planning is the nursing care plan. The nursing orders written on the nursing care plan reflect the objectives which have been formulated, the priorities which have been set, and the approaches which have been selected, as well as the actions delegated to nursing by other members of the health team. The nursing care plan gives a picture of the total nursing care of the patient. Too many so-called nursing care plans

[6]Mary B. Tarasuk, *et al.*, "An Experimental Test of the Importance of Communication Skills for Effective Nursing," *Social Interaction and Patient Care*, James K. Skipper and Robert C. Leonard, eds. (Philadelphia: J. B. Lippincott Co., 1965), pp. 110-120.

merely itemize those measures the physician has delegated to the nurse, with little or no evidence of independent nursing care.

If the assessment of the patient has been carefully done and the patient's problem identified, there should be some assurance that the nursing care plan is complete, that it meets the essential nursing needs of the patient. However. if the author's observations are a representative sample of general practice, it may not be valid to assume that either a careful assessment or a complete nursing care plan is the usual pattern of nursing practice. It seems advisable that there be some scheme so that no essential aspect of care is overlooked. One way to do this is to correlate the general categories of assessment data with the categories of the nursing care plan. For instance, there might be space allocated on the nursing care plan for each of the patterns of functioning to remind the nurse to write nursing orders in those categories which apply to the individual patient.

Some forms for nursing care plans use so much space for detailed activities that little space is left for nursing objectives and independent nursing actions. Creativity and initiative may thus be stifled. Nursing care may be stereotyped. Having a special space for the details of nursing care can force the nurse to think of the patient's needs in these areas. All areas do not necessarily apply to all patients. For instance, one patient may have many teaching needs and hardly any activity needs, whereas the reverse might be true for another patient. One space will be jammed with nursing orders, the other practically blank. This might mean that the full space would be difficult to read. A nursing care plan must be legible if it is to be used by nursing personnel.

Instead of a detailed format for the nursing care plan, one with general categories and little detail may be preferred. One way to assure completeness when a nondetailed format is used is to have a card from a card file or a page of a pocket-notebook to which the nurse can refer as a reminder of all possible needs of the patient. This method allows for more flexibility in using space on the care plan, space which can be used for nursing orders pertaining to the patient's particular problems. With this system, little or no space is given to areas in which the patient is self-sufficient, and enough space is available for those aspects of nursing care needed.

Content of the Care Plan

Most formats for nursing care plans are divided into several sections, the titles and details of each section differing in various agencies. One section of the nursing care plan is the general care section which lists items of care common to many patients. What is included in this section will vary with the type of patients cared for by the agency or by the unit within the agency. Listing items of general care serves as a reminder of these aspects of care. Following are some of the items which might be listed in a general care section for hospitalized patients and the nature of the nursing orders pertaining to each item.

bath—type, time, special adaptations
oral hygiene—type, time, special adaptations, denture care, brand of dentifrice and mouth wash preferred
diet—type, time of serving other than usual, need for assistance, and other adaptations
fluids—amount indicated, type preferred or prescribed, spacing of intake over time period, other adaptations
intake and output—frequency of measuring
elimination—special problems, observations, assistance needed
activity—type, amount, assistance needed, handicap, prostheses, frequency of turning, and range of motion exercises
rest/sleep—nap times, bedtime rituals, hour of retiring, arising
diversion—preferences, hobbies, visitors
vital signs—type, frequency, adaptations, who to notify if significant changes occur, what changes are significant if different from what is ordinarily considered important

In specialized units, there may be other items which might be added to the general care section. On an obstetrical unit, a place is designated for postpartum checks and infant feeding schedule. On a coronary care unit, the care plan form may have space for indicating the frequency of electrocardiogram write-outs and for the dosage and method of administration of oxygen. A rehabilitation unit might include more detail on the activities of daily living, promotion of self-help, positioning devices.

A section of the nursing care plan should list the patient's appointments since this information is vital to coordinating his care. The time he spends in rehabilitation service, the radiotherapy department, or other place is recorded. Any diagnostic tests or therapeutic measures which may affect nursing care or which should be considered in coordinating his care may be listed in this section.

Medicine and treatment section of the nursing care plan will itemize drugs the patient receives, dosage, time and method of administration, and the types and timing of treatments. Both scheduled and P.R.N. medications and treatments should be included. This section should include any adaptations to the patient in methods of administration of the drug, whether or not an oral medication is diluted, if tablets are crushed, the order in which the patient wishes to take the medications if this is important to him. For injections, any adaptations in needle size or site of injection should be noted. Results to be noted and reported, possible side and toxic effects to observe can be recorded in this section.

The section of the nursing care plan devoted to independent nursing measures should list the nursing objectives, ranked according to priority, and the nursing actions selected to achieve each objective. It may be desirable to state both the problem and the objective in one column and the nursing actions opposite these in another column.

Because the condition of the patient is seldom static, his needs for nursing care change frequently. Changes in the physician's plan of therapy necessitate revisions of the nursing care plan. The nursing care plan must coincide with the patient's changing status. There is nothing that dissuades nursing personnel from using a nursing care plan more than one which is out of date. An out-of-date care plan is a meaningless, useless form. To keep the nursing care plan current requires a concerted effort, especially among nurse-team leaders. There are a number of ways of doing this. The team leader might set aside a certain time each day (or longer interval in some instances) for quickly reviewing the nursing care plans of her group of patients and changing those nursing orders which need changing. If the team leader carries the *Kardex* file of nursing care plans with her when she makes rounds to see her patients, she can check the care plan as she visits each patient and can either note or actually make needed changes. The exchange-of-shift report or the team conference is suitable for reviewing nursing care plans and up-dating them.

The practice of erasing items and replacing them with new nursing orders makes it awkward to use the nursing care plan as a research tool. Yet the information on care plans could be a valuable source of data for nursing research. Nursing care plans usually are not part of the patient's permanent medical record. If the profession of nursing is to grow and develop, there must be some way of studying in depth the objectives for patient care devised by nurses and the nursing actions they design and the results of those actions. Unless a record is kept of this information, all of it is lost to the advancement of nursing. One solution might be "progress notes" in each patient's record where the changes made in the nursing care plan and the reasons for the changes are recorded.

Discharge Plans

Professional nursing should aim at providing continuity of care for the patient. It is too late to plan for this on the day a patient is transferred or dismissed. The nursing care plan should reflect not only the nursing needs of the patient in the present facility but those needs related to his transition to another agency or his home. This aspect of the nursing care plan is sometimes called a discharge plan. When the patient moves within an agency, from agency to agency, or from agency to home or home back to agency, his nursing care should continue uninterrupted. The discharge portion of the nursing care plan is a bridge between two environments and should reflect the adjustments the patient, his family, or the new caretakers will need to make to the new situation. The plan should indicate how the nurse can facilitate the transition. Nursing actions may include teaching, referring, supervising the patient or family in practicing some aspect of care.

Date	MEDICATIONS		Date	P.R.N. MEDICATIONS
11/17	Colace 100mg	8 - 8	11/17	Morphine Sulf. 15mg (H) q 3-4 h.
11/17	Phenobarbital 15mg	8 - 2 - 8		p.r.n. for chest pain.
11/17	Milk of Magnesia 30ml	8p	11/17	Tuinal 100mg H.S. prn sleep
11/17	Atropine 0.4 mg p.o.	6 - 2 - 10		
				APPOINTMENTS
			11/18	SGOT, CPK, LDH daily x 3 11/18, 19, 20
			11/18	ECG daily x 3 11/18, 19, 20
	ALLERGIES none known			

C---- Mr. L.

Date	NURSING PROBLEMS & OBJECTIVES	APPROACHES
11/17	Ineffectual circulation -	Explain care as given.
	Mr C will develop no major arrhythmias	Recognize his efforts to relax
		No very hot or cold foods or liquids.
		No rectal exams or treatments
		Instruct to breathe through mouth and
		not strain when turning, having B.M.
		Instruct visitors to avoid topics known to
		upset him. Screen T.V., radio, visitors
		- no excitement
		Listen & reflect as he verbalizes his concerns
	Mr C. will have a suitable home	Help re-establish a daily schedule
	program	Listen & explore changes in life pattern
		Instruct in post-MI exercise program,
		diet, follow-up. Adjust to his likes
		Foster interest in his coin collection.

Figure 5.1. Nursing Care for Mr. L. C.

Nurses in the present agency and the next should be aware of the total plan of care for the patient and the part they play in accomplishing the goals. When a patient is transferred from one facility to another, a written resumé of his nursing care should accompany him. Continuity of care requires that there be communication between nurses in various agencies, community health nurses, and family members. This communication is essential for the evaluation of nursing care so that nurses in each facility can profit from the other's experience with the patient.

NURSING CARE PLAN

Date	GENERAL CARE	
	GENERAL CARE	(Rt.), L. Handed
11/18 LVN.	Personal Hygiene--Bath @ H.S.	Shampoo defer
LVN.	Oral Hygiene Colgate's. Brush Teeth after breakfast & supper	
LVN	Skin Care Back rub 10 am + H.S.	Shave after breakfast
	Food & Fluids--Diet Soft. 1500 cal 500 mg Na	Feed wife or aide
	Fluids 1500 ml/day 800 ml/a.m. 500 ml/p.m. 200 ml/noc	Intake 8 hr totals
	Elimination--Urine Urinal - keep in easy reach	Output 8 hr totals
RN	Bowels Assist to commode - No straining. If constipated - report to Dr.	
	Exercise—Walk none - Bed rest	Turn may Turn self.
	Position Head of bed elevated > 20°	ROM passive - arms, legs X5 8-12-4-8
LVN.	Rest/Sleep Bathe at H.S. Give Bible to read. Quiet time 10 am-12, 4-6 pm	
	Diversion Radio. Nurses. Wife - daughter visit	
RN.	Note & Record: Temp. 4pm. 8pm. Pulse apical + Pulse Deficit q 2 h	Resp. q 2 h - even hour
	B.P. q 2 h. even hour C.V.P.	Weight
	Rhythm strips 8-12-4-8-12-4	

		Date	TREATMENTS
11/18 LVN.	Replace electrodes - day - 10a.	11/17	O_2 - nasal prongs. 3 L/min
11/18 LVN	Deep breathing ex. X10 - 8-12-4-8	11/17	IV. D5W 10-12 minidrops/min.
11/18	Foot board.	11/17	Parker-Davis elastic Stockings
A	Likes to eat one food at a time - let him select order of eating.		
11/18 LVN	Remove and replace elastic stockings 6a - 2 - 10p.		

Next of Kin Wife, Mrs Vera 795-4321 Diagnosis Ant. Myocardial Infarction
Religion Baptist Surgery
Name C...., Mr L... Age 64 Case No. 15-20-72 Dr. R.J.

Figure 5.1. (Continued)

On the other hand, for a patient who frequently transfers between agencies and home, there is always the possibility that his care might become stereotyped. Nurses in the various settings might rely on the assessment and planning made by their counterparts in another agency and fail to see the patient's true needs. From time to time it pays to take a fresh look at such a patient—or any patient, for that matter—to see whether his needs are in fact being gratified.

* * * *

Date	MEDICATIONS	Date	P.R.N. MEDICATIONS
11/24	Dulcolax Supp 8^{30} a	11/23	Demerol 75 mg (M) q 3-4 hrs
			p.r.n. post. op. pain.
			APPOINTMENTS
ALLERGIES none known			

B.... Mr. A.

Date	NURSING PROBLEMS & OBJECTIVES	APPROACHES
11/25	Immobility + paraplegia - Mr B will be able to	
	— transfer self from bed → wheelchair → bed	Trapeze exercises for arms 8-12-4-8
	—	Consult c̄ P.T. re. weight lifting (later)
		Shift weight to relieve pressure when
		in bed or wh ch.
		Practice transfer activities after recovery
		from operation.
	- Control bowels + bladder	Bladder control deferred -
		Supp. + bedpan at usual time for Bm.
		Instruct re: supp insertion + sensory
		stimulation of anal area. Practice later
	- have a daily home schedule.	Talk c̄ re: home schedule.
		Re-establish daily schedule.
	- have plans for employment	Explore interests re: employment, decision
		Refer to voc. rehab.
		Have Mrs. B. explore community facilities

Figure 5.2. Nursing Care Plan for Mr. A. B.

Not all nursing care performed for the patient is derived from orders written on the nursing care plan. There are many on-the-spot situations in which the nurse must assess, plan, act, and evaluate spontaneously. If such situations are likely to be repeated for the patient, then her actions should become a part of the nursing care plan. If a repeat occurrence is unlikely, there is no need to add this information to the nursing care plan. It will, of course, be included in the permanent record of the patient.

Essential to the implementation of a nursing care plan is the ability of the nurse to write unambiguous nursing orders.

NURSING CARE PLAN

Date	GENERAL CARE
	(Rt.), L. Handed
11/25.	Personal Hygiene--Bath H.S. — Shampoo q. Wed.
	5 Oral Hygiene Crest. Brush teeth after breakfast & H.S.
	Skin Care massage & lotion to back q2h. 8-10-12-2-4-6 etc. Shave in am.
	Food & Fluids--Diet Surg. liquids — Feed Straw for drinking
	Fluids IV. As soon as tolerated - 3000 ml/day — Intake 8 hr totals
	Elimination--Urine Foley c̄ G.U. Irrigant @ 12 drops/min — Output 8 hr totals
	Bowels Place on fracture pan 30 min after supp.
	Exercise--Walk CircOlectric bed - bed rest — Turn q 2 hrs. 8-10-12 etc.
	Position L side → prone → supine — ROM passive to legs each time turned
	Rest/Sleep 2 blankets - Have room as dark and quiet as possible
	Diversion Find out what interests him.
	Note & Record: Temp. 8-12-4-8-12 Pulse q 2 hrs - even hrs. Resp. q 2 h.
	B.P. q 2 hr. - even hrs C.V.P. — Weight
	Check legs for motion, sensation 6-10-6-10 Report change to T.L.
	Inspect skin daily during bath for redness, irritation
	Check position for proper alignment each time care is given.

Date		Date	TREATMENTS
11/24.	10 deep breaths, 2-3 coughs q 2 h - even hours.	11/23	IPPB 5 min c̄ N.S. 8a. 2-10pm. I.T.
	Footboard -	11/23	No movement of trunk while doing R.O.M.
	Heels off mattress at all times		
	Log roll when turning	11/25	PT. begin instruction in conditioning exercises.
	Explain hospital routines and all care given.		
	Explore his thoughts re: condition etc		
	Cath care (wash & apply neo-sporin to meatus 6a. 2-10 p.m.		

Next of Kin wife - Mrs Nancy 415-9876 — Diagnosis Cord Injury T 10-11 Nov. 22
Religion none — Surgery Decompression laminectomy 11/23
Name B... Mr. A. — Age 29 Case No. 19-20-21 Dr. L.D.

Figure 5.2. (Continued)

Writing Nursing Orders

To implement the selected approaches to the various problems of the patient, nursing orders must be written into the nursing care plan. These are the directives for the nursing actions to be carried out. These written orders are one way of communicating to all personnel giving nursing care. They should give some assurance that care is consistently carried out by all nurses on all shifts and from day to day or contact to contact. In order for the directives to be followed consistently and uniformly, they should be written in specific terms which have a minimal possibility for misinterpretation. The words used should accurately describe the nursing actions envisioned by the nurses who planned the care. Action verbs which precisely describe the desired nursing action should be used.

Objective description of nursing actions is not an easy task. Some actions are very straight-forward; others are more elusive, some are unique to the nurse's own personality; some can be repeated with ease by many nursing personnel, some are difficult to duplicate. Obviously, it is simpler to have uniformity of action in the manual skills than in the interpersonal skills. Furthermore, uniformity may be highly desirable for some nursing actions, whereas uniformity of interpersonal techniques could suppress the individuality of the nurse. If nursing is to develop as a profession, there must be a way to describe interpersonal skills precisely enough so that the method can be adapted by different nurses who interact with a given patient and so that all achieve the desired end. Only by precise description of nursing actions will the profession be able to predict that a specific nursing action has a high probability of achieving the desired result.

Two nurse leaders who have contributed much to the description of what goes on between nurses and patients, even though their views differ, are Peplau[7] and Orlando[8]. There are several schools of thought, each explaining the dynamics of human relationships in different ways. Because of the different approaches to interpersonal relationships advocated by diverse authorities, the nurse will prescribe interpersonal nursing actions within her own frame of reference. When a satisfactory approach is discovered for helping a patient deal with an emotional problem, this approach could be discussed in a team conference and then written as a nursing order in such a way that all will understand the approach. Role-playing a typical interaction during a team conference is one way to help the nursing team members understand their role in the prescribed interaction.

One common nursing order is "give emotional support." How this order is carried out is probably as variable as the number of nurses attending the patient. What the person needs and desires in the way of emotional support should be specified. Nursing orders might be patterned after the operational definitions of the particular emotional problem the patient has, such as anxiety, anger, or manipulative behavior.[9]

Another common ineffective nursing order is "Encourage fluids." This order is ambiguous, indefinite, and perfunctory. No quantity is specified,

---

7Hildegard Peplau, "Talking with Patients," *American Journal of Nursing* 60:7 (1960):964-6; Hildegard Peplau, *Interpersonal Relations in Nursing* (New York: J. P. Putnam's Sons, 1952).

8Ida Jean Orlando, *The Dynamic Nurse-Patient Relationship* (New York: G. P. Putnam's Sons, 1961).

9Shirley F. Burd and Margaret A. Marshall (eds.), *Some Clinical Approaches to Psychiatric Nursing* (New York: The Macmillan Co., 1963), pp.110-115, 116-124, 323-7.

one nurse might interpret this as 1000 ml., another as 3000 ml. If a person needs fluids he must drink them, not merely be "encouraged" to drink them. The order could read "Give 200 ml. fluids (may specify type if this makes a difference) at 8, 10 a.m., 2, 4, 8, 10 p.m. To reiterate, in order to write nursing orders which communicate the intent of those who plan nursing care, the nurse's actions must be described in words which clearly express that intent.

Some nursing orders relate to observation of the patient's behavior, symptoms, signs, and reactions. While observation is largely a function of assessment, observation and intervention so closely follow each other in time that it is often hard to separate them. Both the assessment and the intervention, even the evaluation, may be included in one nurse-patient contact. Once the initial assessment has been made, it is essential that the nurse decide what on-going observations pertain to the patient's condition and the frequency of the observations. Decisions regarding the type and frequency of the on-going appraisal are a part of planning. Whatever the nurse decides are essential on-going observations should be written as nursing orders on the nursing care plan. Combined with this order is the appropriate intervention, what to do if significant changes occur. It may be desirable to include in the order what the significant changes are, to whom to report the changes, and any other appropriate action. The intervention arising from many observations made by nurses is just to record and/or report the information. If the observation shows that the patient has no problem, conveying this information to the patient or health team members may be all the intervention that is required. To illustrate the need for indicating what changes are significant, consider this example. It is common practice for nurses to notify the physician if a patient's blood pressure drops below 90 mm. of mercury. If a patient's usual blood pressure is 180/120 it could be disastrous to the patient (to say nothing of the nurse!) to let this patient's pressure drop to a systolic of 90 mm. of mercury without notifying the physician. The nursing order, then, would include the times to check the blood pressure and to report a systolic of less than 160 mm. or more than 200 mm. of mercury to the team leader.

Some nursing orders might direct the nurse to report the presence or absence of some sign or symptom. The following example of a nursing order relates to edema. "Check sacral area and feet for edema—report presence or absence to team leader, chart findings." From the foregoing examples it can be seen that assessment and intervention may be closely intertwined and one nursing order may cover both assessment and intervention.

Each nursing order consists of four parts which answer the four questions: What? When? How? Who?

What refers to the actual nursing measure planned for the patient, usually preceded by the action verb which specifies the nature of the action. Some of these action verbs are Teach .... Listen .... Refer to .... Give .... Feed .... Walk .... Take to .... Report .... Report immediately ....

When will indicate the timing and frequency of the activity. In practical experience, it is more satisfactory to indicate specific hours for an action to be carried out than to use such nonspecifics as B.I.D., once a shift, once daily, or q4h. A B.I.D. order could be done at the end of one shift and the beginning of the next, the spacing thereby decreasing the effectiveness of the action. "Once daily" orders may easily be relegated to another shift by a busy nurse, thus interfering with the total program of the patient or nursing team. Or the fact that the measure was not carried out may not be communicated at the exchange-of-shift report, leaving it not done at all.

If the nurse-leader who writes the nursing orders is specific and careful in writing times, a great deal will be accomplished toward organizing the patient's schedule and the work of the nursing team. She can assign times in such a way as to cluster appropriate activities together, thereby assuring maximum utilization of each nurse-patient encounter. Moreover, assigning specific times can do much toward spacing team activities evenly throughout the day rather than in such large clusters that it is impossible to get everything done on time.

How indicates the way the measure is adapted to the individual patient. Any adaptation of personal hygiene measures, general nursing procedures, and treatments should be specified. If a measure is carried out in a routine manner, such as that suggested in the procedure manual, there will be no need to include a *How* in the nursing order. It is unfair to a patient for him to have to tell every nurse who cares for him that he likes a certain thing done in a certain way. If he doesn't like to wear his dentures at night, this should be written on the nursing care plan with his other bedtime care so that he will not have to tell this to every nurse. Or, if a patient is catheterized and the nurse learns that a 16F catheter is too large and this size catheter is routinely supplied, the order to catheterize should be qualified to include the need for a 14F catheter. If a patient cannot tolerate "O.K." in the speech of those caring for him, this too should be included in the nursing care plan. To assume that these specifics of care will be passed on by word of mouth is not valid.

Included in the *How* of the order should be an indication or the amount of assistance the patient needs to help himself: whether he is totally reliant on the nurse for the needed care, if he only needs supplies placed within easy reach, if he needs some specific assistance but is otherwise self-reliant or is entirely self-reliant. In the clinical situation, a graded scale using letters or symbols can be utilized on the nursing care plan to indicate how much help the patient needs. This scale should be understood by all who refer to the nursing care plan. For instance, *T* might mean total care; S, provide supplies; *A*, assist (and specify what kind of assistance); *I*, independent. For a nursing order regarding a bed bath, a *T* with the order would indicate that the nurse give the bed bath without any self-help by the patient; an *S* that the nurse provides supplies and the patient can give his own bath; an *SA* that supplies must be provided and the patient needs help with bathing back and legs; an *I* that the patient can get his own supplies and give his own bath.

Who should indicate the title of the nursing team member responsible for carrying out the particular activity. This can be done by placing abbreviations of the title opposite each order, such as *T.L.* for team leader, *R.N.* for staff nurse, *L.V.N.* or *L.P.N.* for the licensed vocational nurse, *A* for nursing assistants. Some other system might be devised by the agency.

When the nursing order indicates the type of team member best able to carry out the order, a quick perusal of nursing care plans can lead to a reasonable estimate of staffing needs. This information is valuable in the work planning conference for the team so that nursing activities can be quickly assigned to the various team members. The team member can know what aspect of the care (one item or total care) of each patient is her responsibility. Specific nursing orders which include the *what, when,* and *by whom* aspects for a group of patients could be processed by a computer in order to facilitate the planning of the work for the team.

In order to assign team members to the tasks they can do best, the team leader should have a basic understanding of the abilities and preparation of each level of nursing personnel. In addition, she should be familiar with the strengths and deficiencies of individual workers. As stated in Chapter 2, there are no distinct lines separating the knowledge and performance of the different levels of nursing personnel. How well the individual performs ranges over rather wide norms since performance depends not only on differences in education but also on differences in ability, motivation, and other characteristics. The team leader must acquaint herself with the particular strengths and weaknesses of the individual nurses with whom she works. On this basis, she assigns them to the tasks at hand.

Some examples of nursing orders which might be written to adapt general care to an individual patient are indicated in Table 5.2. Those items in parentheses would be ordered by the physician.

* * * *

The planning phase of nursing intervention is never-ending, the dynamics of the person's health/illness status demand continuous planning so that nursing care equilibrates with the patient's needs. Planning is an essential component of professional nursing. It gives goal-direction to what is done for the patient. It requires the best intellectual efforts of a skillful, knowledgeable nurse.

Table 5.2
Examples of Nursing Orders

Item	Assistance needed	Nursing Order	Worker
Bath	T	Full bath before breakfast M.W.F. Partial bath before breakfast S.T.Th.S.	L.V.N.
oral hygiene	S	Colgate's toothpaste, Scope mouthwash. After breakfast, and H.S.	L.V.N.
diet	S	(soft diet/1200 cal.) cut meat in bite-size, pour drinks, give straw. Main meal @ noon.	A.
		Teach re: 1200 cal. diet.	R.N.
Fluids	S	(1500 ml/day) 800 ml/a.m., 500 ml/p.m., 200 ml/noc. Give orange juice @ 10 a.m., pine-apple or apple juice @ 4 p.m., 200 ml. Give straw for drinking	A.
Intake and Output	T	Accurate. Total @ 2 p.m., 10 p.m., 6 a.m. Weight @ 6 a.m., MWF.	L.V.N.
Elimination	S	Note and report urgency or stress incontinence. If no B.M. by 8 p.m., give p.r.n. laxative. Put on bedpan for B.M. after breakfast.	L.V.N.
Rest/sleep	S	Hot cocoa, 200 ml. @ H.S. – 10 p.m. Turn pillow radio to music station. Give him his devotional book to read. Special massage to back and neck. Undisturbed for nap—11 a.m.-12, 4-5 p.m.	L.V.N.
Activity	S	ROM x 10 @ 8 a.m., 1, 4, p.m. H.S. Remind to exercise feet and legs each time care is given. Can turn self.	
Diversion	S	Offer books P.R.N. Ask volunteer to obtain books from cart. Find another pt. to play checkers with him P.R.N.— Visitors ad. lib.	A.
		Business associates (Mr. S. G. and Mr. H. K. to stay only 5 min. Remind them to avoid discussing worrisome problems.	R.N.
Vital signs	T	T @ 4 p.m., 8 p.m. P.R., B.P. 8, 12, 4, 8 and when awake during noc. Take B.P. on left arm. Report to T.L. pulse > 100 or < 60, B.P. > 180 or <100.	L.V.N.

REFERENCES

*BAIN, BARBARA, and BAILEY, JANE. "How a Communication Tool Led to the Development of a Nursing Care Plan." *Nursing Outlook* 15:10(1967): 48-51.

*BURGESS, MIRIAM G. "A Nursing Care Plan for the Postoperative Patient in the Recovery Room and Intensive Care Unit." *Nursing Clinics of North America* 3:3(1968):499-502.

*BUTTS, CLARENCE L. and CANNEY, VESTA E. "The Unresponsive Patient." *American Journal of Nursing* 67:9(1967):1886-8.

*DAVID, JANIS H. *et al. Guidelines for Discharge Planning.* Downey, Calif.: Attending Staff Association of Rancho Los Amigos Hospital, Inc. 1968.

DUNCAN, A. R. C. "Techniques of Decision Making." *Readings in Management,* Ernest Dale (ed.). New York: McGraw-Hill Book Company, 387-93, 1965.

*HARRISON, CHERIE. "Deliberative Nursing Process versus Automatic Nurse Action." *Nursing Clinics of North America* 1:3(1966):387-97.

KELLY, NANCY C. "Nursing Care Plans." *Nursing Outlook* 14:5(1966):61-4.

MAGER, ROBERT. *Preparing Instructional Objectives.* Palo Alto, Calif.: Fearon Publishers, Inc. 1962.

MANSFIELD, ELAINE. "Use of Patient Care Plans by Aides." *Nursing Outlook* 15:4(1967):72-4.

*MATTHIESEN, JANICE E. "Tommy Had Leukemia." *American Journal of Nursing* 68:11(1968):2408-12.

*McDONALD, FREDERICK J. and HARMS, MARY T. "Theoretical Model for an Experimental Curriculum." *Nursing Outlook* 14:8(1966):48-51.

NEWMAN, WILLIAM H. and SUMMER, CHARLES E. JR. *The Process of Management.* Englewood Cliffs: Prentice-Hall, Inc. 1963.

ORLANDO, IDA JEAN. *The Dynamic Nurse-Patient Relationship.* New York: G. P. Putnam's Sons, 1961.

*PEABODY, SYLVIA A. "Assessment and Planning for Continuity of Care." *Nursing Clinics of North America* 4:2(1969):303-10.

PEPLAU, HILDEGARD E. "Talking with Patients." *American Journal of Nursing* 60:7(1960):964-6.

*TARASUK, MARY B. *et al.* "An Experimental Test of the Importance of Communication Skills for Effective Nursing." *Social Interaction and Patient Care.* James K. Skipper and Robert C. Leonard. (eds.) Philadelphia: J. B. Lippincott. 110-20, 1965.

*WAGNER, BERNIECE M. "Care Plans—Right, Reasonable, and Reachable." *American Journal of Nursing* 69:5(1969):986-90.

CLINICAL EXPERIENCE

1. Select two or three problems you have identified for patients. Follow through the planning steps: formulate objectives; design alternative approaches and select one based on its probability of success and desirability; write appropriate nursing orders on the nursing care plan.
2. Conduct a team conference with and without the patient present. Present a high priority or difficult nursing problem to the group and have the group work through the planning steps. Compare the results when the patient is or is not included.

*Suggested for additional reading.

3. Work through the planning steps of one nursing problem for a patient by yourself. Conduct a team conference regarding the same nursing problem. Compare the results of individual and group planning.
4. Consult with a clinical specialist regarding a nursing problem in the area of her expertise. Critically examine the nursing orders which the clinical specialist writes.
5. Compare the specificity of nursing orders written to meet physical needs with those written to meet emotional, spiritual, or social needs. Discuss with others ways of writing more specific orders for emotional, spiritual, or social needs.

Chapter 6

Intervention—Nursing Action

Indirect, away-from-the-patient nursing intervention has been described as planning. The doing-interacting, direct, with-the-patient nursing intervention will be described as nursing action. Nursing actions comprise what the nurse does for, with, and to a patient in order to achieve nursing objectives. The operation and manipulation of therapeutic devices and the administration of medications and treatments constitute some nursing actions. Most of these are dependent nursing actions prescribed by physicians or other members of the health team and carried out by the nurse. Of equal or greater concern to the nurse are independent nursing actions—those designed and carried out by nurses to meet the nursing needs of people. Most of the independent nursing actions are either a "laying on of hands" or communication. Nursing actions are interpersonal; they take place between persons, between the nurse and the patient, the family, or the people in a community.

The philosophy of nursing to which a nurse subscribes will determine the types of nursing actions she uses in meeting the needs of her patients. Philosophy will dictate what and how much a nurse teaches a patient, the types of patient problems with which she will counsel the patient, what she sees as dependent and independent nursing action, or whether she deals with future needs of the patient as well as the here-and-now. Institutional policy and availability of supplies and equipment will also determine the types of nursing action used. Policy may state that the physical therapist rather than the nurse gives some kinds of exercise; it may distinguish between the diet teaching done by the nurse and the dietitian, or it may or may not allow the nurse to give intravenous injections. Available equipment and supplies limit or expand nursing actions. The development of electronic monitoring equipment has changed what a nurse does with the critically ill. Whether a hypothermia unit is available may determine what cooling measures are used to reduce a fever. If closed circuit television is available, the nurse might find this a valuable teaching tool.

The nurse's own capabilities are another determinant of nursing action —what she does or does not know how to do, the kinds of communication with which she feels comfortable, and the nonverbal communication characteristic of her personality. One nurse may feel comfortable holding a patient's hand to communicate her interest and concern for the patient's distress; another nurse might see this as inappropriate and an ineffective form of communication for her. The nurse is unlikely to attempt a nursing action with which she is unfamiliar; it would be difficult to imagine a nurse giving effective cardiopulmonary resuscitation if she had never learned how to do this, or a nurse attempting to teach a patient how to give his own insulin if she were not competent in the administration of insulin. Two points might be interjected here: one, the nurse who attempts a nursing action she is not qualified to perform safely is liable for malpractice; the other, the nurse is obligated to society to continue to learn new nursing actions as new knowledge and equipment become available.

Nursing actions test the hypotheses posed in the planning stage. When alternative courses of action were considered, it was hypothesized that the one selected would have a good chance of achieving the nursing objective. Actually trying out the proposed nursing action with the patient, and evaluating its effectiveness, tests the hypothesis. If the action contributes to the objective, the action is incorporated into the nursing care plan as an appropriate approach to the patient's problem. If the action is ineffective, the approach will be rejected in favor of another one.

TYPES OF NURSING ACTION

"Laying-on-of-hands" type of nursing actions provides comfort, support, therapy, and protection for the patient. This type of nursing action is typical of the personal service and technical roles of the nurse, the caring and curing components of nursing.

Nursing actions requiring the "laying on of hands" are often delegated to the nonprofessional nurse or the nursing assistant. In delegating these functions to others, the professional nurse loses some opportunities to communicate nonverbally with the patient and to demonstrate her "caring" by actions which might build the confidence of the patient in the nurse's professional competence. The doing of these nursing acts for and with the patient is one way to establish rapport with him and help him feel that he can trust the nurse.

The "laying on of hands" offers as many opportunities for applying scientific principles to patient care as any other type of nursing action. It is important that professional nurses initiate research into the physiological and psychological effects of these actions. The validity of many traditional nursing actions must be substantiated by research if the profession of nursing is to have a sound scientific base. To illustrate, positioning a patient requires the "laying on of hands." Nurses use position and exercise for the comfort of the patient, for the prevention of the complications of inactivity, for rehabilitation, and to obtain a desired physiological effect. How often does the nurse know that the position achieved the desired effect? Does she know that a selected position may or may not alter the patient's physiology in a beneficial way? It may be an intuitive act to place a dyspneic patient in a sitting position. On the other hand, purposeful positioning probably can influence other body functions more than nurses realize. Position is one determinant of venous return, therefore, of cardiac output. Position is one factor in kidney function. The excretion of certain electrolytes is altered by position change. Position affects blood pressure and the distribution of blood to certain body parts. Position alters the rate of production of some hormones. Position influences the motility and emptying of various sections of the gastrointestinal tract. Position determines the amount of drainage from a body cavity or abscess and the spread of infectious material from one part of the body to another. A change in position may relieve pain. Professional nurses working directly with patients can ask researchable questions regarding the measurable effects of nursing actions on patients. Nursing research might well aim to find out new ways in which nurses can use position or other independent nursing actions to achieve desired physiologic effects.

Caring and curing components of nursing practice which relieve symptoms such as pain, nausea, cough, fever, edema, and insomnia initiate a variety of nursing actions. The supporting hand, the placing of a cool compress on a fevered brow, positioning edematous parts, the back rub to induce relaxation and sleep, placing a pillow to provide support and comfort are all simple nursing actions which may relieve discomforts. Hopefully these independent nursing actions are considered as alternatives to giving prescribed medication to relieve symptoms. The specific effects of certain nursing actions on the relief of symptoms is another area wide open to nursing research. Unless professional nurses are involved in using these nursing actions to accomplish specific purposes, they are not apt to ask the questions nor to have the hunches which stimulate research. From this kind of research will come an identifiable body of knowledge essential to the practice of nursing.

Many nursing actions utilize communication as the mode of nursing therapy. In the nurse-patient relationship the purpose of communication may be to teach, counsel, socialize, obtain information, or show interest and concern. All of these are independent nursing actions. Communication is used in all of the roles of nursing and in each of the care, cure, coordination components of nursing. The nurse uses herself as a therapeutic agent when she employs communication as a nursing action. Not only speaking, but listening, posture, general appearance, facial expression, gestures, the distance between the nurse and the patient, the use of touch—all a part of the nurse's personality—are used to communicate.

Language is a very commonly used medium of communication and its importance in the nurse-patient relationship should not be underestimated. Some forms of nonverbal communication have special significance for nursing because of the interpersonal nature of nursing. Several references at the end of this chapter refer to touch, space, and distance as worthy of consideration in the planning of patient care. When the nurse uses these nonverbal forms of communication as nursing actions, the communication cycle must be completed by feedback from the receiver. Certainly the nurse must be aware of the meanings of these forms of communication so that she will use them to convey the intended message. As with many other concepts, nursing research is needed to specify the meanings of touch, space, and distance in the nurse-patient relationship and their use as purposeful nursing actions.

ACTIONS RELATED TO THE COMPONENTS OF WHOLENESS

To every nursing action, the patient responds as a whole; his reactions involve all of the components of wholeness. An action may be primarily designed to help solve a physical or an emotional problem, but the response is holistic—what is done to the part affects the whole. It is a paradox to describe nursing actions as affecting any one dimension of the whole, but some typical nursing actions will be presented in this way to remind the nurse of the wide possibility of independent nursing actions available to her. Yet the nurse must ever keep in mind the holistic effects of each nursing action. By doing so, she may use one nursing action to contribute to several nursing objectives.

Actions to Meet Physical Needs

Many of the nursing actions performed to meet physical needs involve the "laying on of hands." They are concerned with personal hygiene, activities of daily living, measures to relieve symptoms and maintain the patient's optimal patterns of functioning. In addition, communication skills are used to counsel the patient regarding physical problems and to teach him how to maintain his patterns of functioning in the most healthful manner or how to adapt his usual patterns to a therapeutic or rehabilitation program.

Actions to Meet Intellectual Needs

When a person is physically or mentally ill, his mind may not function in a normal way or he may not be able to meet the need for intellectual stimulation which is conducive to health of mind. Illness may interfere with a person's ability to learn, with the result that the nurse may have to explain the same thing to him several times. Likewise, a background of poverty and deprivation may interfere with a person's ability to learn. With due consideration for the patient's background and for his state of health or illness, nursing care should include intellectual stimulation for the patient. Intellectual stimulation may mean explaining to him various aspects of his program, teaching him what he wants to learn, or helping him find a community facility to teach him. It could be providing him with newspapers or magazines, radio or television. Friends and family may be enlisted to provide the intellectual stimulation needed by the patient.

Illness and the sensory deprivation accompanying illness may interfere with a person's ability to concentrate, to solve problems. If the condition is temporary, due to the stage of illness in which the person is, learning and problem-solving may be delayed until the person is ready. Some type of stimulation through one or more sensory mechanisms is necessary in order to keep the person in touch with reality; this may include providing calendar, clock, simple explanation of ongoing procedures, just saying "This is Monday," "This is your breakfast." Another way of encouraging mental activity is to have the patient make an uncomplicated decision, "Do you want your bath before or after your breakfast?" If the condition is more permanent as with senility, the patient may be confronted with learning and problem-solving tasks appropriate to his level of functioning. It is possible that this practice may retard further regression.

Actions to Meet Emotional Needs

Nursing actions to help the person cope with emotional problems mostly fall within the realm of communication, yet measures to relieve physical discomforts causing and/or resulting from the emotions are indicated. If a patient is experiencing pain and is crying and upset, one approach to the emotional reaction is to relieve the pain. Often, the unknown is a cause for such emotions as fear, withdrawal, or anger. To discuss with the patient what is known about the "unknown" he faces may be comforting. If a preoperative patient expresses fear, talking about the experience, explaining what the experience usually entails, giving the patient a chance to talk about what, in particular, he fears, can help him cope. There are some emotions too deep, too moving, for a person to talk about, and some people cannot express in words their true feelings. The care and concern of an interested person is often of more value than anything else. To "be with" the person through the experience, to sit close to him, perhaps hold his hand, is often an appropriate nursing action. A nursing order to sit with a patient after he has been told he has an incurable disease shows insight into the needs of human beings for personal involvement with other human beings.

Most emotional problems call for an interaction between the nurse and the patient. The nurse helps the patient recognize his own behavior as a manifestation of emotion, explore its meaning, and consider alternative, more constructive methods of coping than the patient has been using.

Actions to Meet Spiritual Needs

What does a nurse do to help a person with his spiritual problems? Some nursing actions are based on the emotional responses to spiritual conflict or frustration, and a counseling-type approach is frequently used for such problems. Referrals to a person's accustomed religious counselor may be the preferred nursing action for dealing with some spiritual problems. When a person is unable to carry on some of his usual patterns of worship, assistance by the nurse in reading from devotional books, praying with the patient, discussing religious beliefs, taking him to a hospital chapel or nearby church may be helpful. Considering how a person's religious beliefs and patterns of life affect his usual daily activities and adjusting his program accordingly may prevent or avert some religious problems.

Serious illness and death may initiate a crisis in one's faith. To permit the patient to talk about his doubts and fears, beliefs and meanings about life and death and the hereafter at such a time can strengthen faith and clarify beliefs. The nurse can listen and encourage expression in such a way as to bring spiritual peace and solace to the patient. A health/illness crisis is not a time to advocate changes in the doctrines held by a person nor to argue with him about religious beliefs, but it is a time to strengthen the faith he has.

If a person has no faith and expresses a need for the comfort and solace it provides, the nurse should be able to share her own faith with the patient. This sharing may be a simple outflowing of her own spiritual experience, which, if kept alive and vital, can give hope and strength to the patient. She can assure the patient that he is not alone in his crisis, that he has an all-wise heavenly Father who is aware of his suffering and who is deeply concerned about him. The parable of the prodigal son can help him understand God's love.[1]

There are some patients and nurses who do not have nor wish a deep religious experience. In this event, the individual's right to make this choice must be respected. If a nurse encounters a patient who needs spiritual or emotional help she cannot give, she should feel free to find some other person who can give the needed help.

Nurses help patients solve health/illness problems, whether physical, intellectual, emotional, or spiritual. The nurse does this by listening, by asking appropriate questions, by helping patients identify their own prob-

[1]The Holy Bible, Luke 15:11-32.

lems, by assisting them to devise alternative courses of action. The nurse can encourage patients to try something other than their usual way. She can refer them to other sources of help or she can help them adjust their social environment.

Actions to Meet Social Needs

What can nursing do toward helping patients with social problems? One major contribution of nursing is helping patients with the emotional reactions they have with role change and role acceptance. A counseling approach is the usual nursing action for such problems. Another approach stems from the nurse's knowledge of community resources for helping people. The nurse can acquaint patients and families with these services and how to make use of them.

Adjustments in the way various nursing actions are carried out should be made in terms of the patient's feelings about modesty, privacy, space, and other factors affected by his culture and value system. For hospitalized or home-bound patients the nurse can suggest ways in which family and friends can help the patient maintain his customary roles, accentuate the roles he can keep, and cope with changing those he must relinquish.

The isolation of illness, hospitalization, or disability interrupts a person's social and occupational life. Some of this isolation is unavoidable, but some of it is unnecessary. The nurse must first recognize the behavior peculiar to isolation, and if she has not already taken measures to prevent as much isolation as possible, she should do so. Also she can initiate actions which shorten the isolation or make it more bearable. Visitors, day rooms, radio and television, semiprivate in contrast to private rooms can all be considered as soon as the physical condition of the patient warrants.

Interpersonal problems of patients or among family members which interfere with optimal health may be approached by the nurse with counseling and teaching actions. If the problems are outside the nurse's competence, she will know about those who can help the patient and make the appropriate referrals.

Actions Regarding Environment

Nurses may control the patient's environment by adjusting temperature and humidity for comfort or regulation of body temperature, by initiating antiseptic or sanitary measures to reduce the number or type of microorganisms in the environment, or by limiting or promoting contacts with other persons. Nurses initiate various safety measures designed to protect the patient from injury, infection, disease, or complication. Safety actions range from side rails on a bed to aseptic technique in the treatment of wounds; from isolating a patient with a communicable disease to arranging room furnishings to prevent falls or to adjusting the temperature of a thermal application to prevent burns.

Nurses also may participate in community action programs which are aimed at improving the safety and healthfulness of the environment. Involvement in programs designed to augment the health care of all citizens within a community is a suitable activity for professional nurses.

* * * *

Approaches which nurses can use to help solve the health/illness problems of people embrace a wide range of nursing actions. The foregoing description of nursing actions is suggestive rather than complete. To use nursing actions intelligently, being cognizant of the holistic effects of each action on the person, is a challenge to professional nursing.

REFERENCES

Browse, Norman L. *The Physiology and Pathology of Bed Rest.* Springfield, Ill.: Charles C. Thomas, Publishers. 1965.

Burton, Arthur, and Heller, Louis G. "The Touching of the Body." *Psychoanalytic Review* 51:1(1964):122-34.

*Cashar, Leah, and Dixson, Barbara K. "The Therapeutic Use of Touch." *Journal of Psychiatric Nursing* 5:5(1967):442-51.

*Curtin, B. Colleen, and Reick, Kay L. "Effects of Bodily Positions on the Systolic Blood Pressure Response to Valsalva's Maneuver." *Nursing Research* 18:2(1969):119-23.

*deGroot, William J. "The Advantages and Disadvantages of Various Patient Positions." *Hospital Medicine* 1:3(1964):10-14.

*Johnson, Betty Sue. "The Meaning of Touch in Nursing." *Nursing Outlook* 13:2(1968):59-60.

*Hall, Edward T. *The Hidden Dimension.* New York: Doubleday & Co., Inc., 1966.

*———*The Silent Language.* Greenwich, Conn.: Fawcett Publications, Inc. 1965.

*McCarthy, Rosemary T. "The Metabolic Cost of Maintaining Five Fixed Body Positions." *Nursing Research* 17:6(1968)539:44.

*Minckley, Barbara B. "Physiological Hazards of Position Changes in the Anesthetized Patient." *American Journal of Nursing.* 69:12(1969):2606-11.

*Morley, Wilbur, *et al.* "Crisis: Paradigms of Intervention." *Journal of Psychiatric Nursing* 5:6(1967):531-44.

*Pluckhan, Margaret L. "Space: The Silent Language." *Nursing Forum* VII:4 (1968):386-97.

Ramphal, Marjorie M. "Values of Routines in Nursing." *Nursing Forum* VI:3 (1967)335-40.

Reeder, Sharon R., and Deck, Edith. "Nurses' Participation in a Group Psychotherapeutic Approach to Antepartal Management." *Nursing Forum* II:4 (1963):81-93.

*Risley, Joan. "Nursing Intervention in Depression." *Perspectives in Psychiatric Care* 5:2(1967):65-76.

*Suggested for additional reading.

*RUBIN, REVA. "Maternal Touch." *Nursing Outlook* 11:11(1963):828-31.
*SCHMITT, YVONNE, *et al.* "Armchair Treatment in the Coronary Care Unit: Effect on Blood Pressure and Pulse." *Nursing Research* 18:2(1969):114-8.

CLINICAL EXPERIENCE

1. Use touch as a nursing action in a variety of clinical situations. Compare the feedback received from patients regarding the meaning of the touch. Write nursing orders regarding touch.
2. Try out various positions to see what effect they have on the vital signs of patients. Compare the results from a number of patients who are in a similar clinical status. Write nursing orders pertaining to purposeful positioning.
3. When interviewing patients, sit at varying distances (intimate, personal, social, public) from the patient. Compare the content of the conversations at the different distances. Write nursing orders pertaining to distance and space.
4. Compare the space assigned to individuals in specialized and general care units in the hospital, in private homes of middle-class and poverty families. Can you detect changes in behavior typical of the person's space allotment?
5. Keep track of the number and kinds of nursing objectives you can work on during a patient's "bath time."

*Suggested for additional reading.

Chapter 7

Evaluation

Final step in the nursing process is evaluation. Without this step, the process is incomplete and it is not known whether the nursing actions taken achieved the desired objectives. This step indicates whether the nursing actions supported the hypotheses and should become a part of the nursing care plan. Without evaluation the nurse is operating in the dark, not knowing whether the care given to patients is satisfying their needs.

There are two aspects of evaluation which may be considered. Of prime importance, as it relates to the nursing process, is the evaluation of the effect of nursing care on the patient. Because the nursing care plan is a written reflection of the care given the patient, it is a good administrative practice to evaluate nursing care plans from time to time. Both of these aspects of evaluation are presented in this chapter.

EVALUATION OF PATIENT CARE

Who Evaluates Care?

Evaluation of nursing care is the mutual concern of all members of the health and nursing teams, but primary responsibility for evaluation rests with the nurse who planned the care. The patient and his family must be involved in evaluation; they are the objects of the nursing actions and should have the final word in determining the effectiveness of the care. For subjective symptoms, such as pain, anxiety, and nausea, the patient is the primary source of evaluation. Even though there are physical manifestations of these symptoms, the patient alone is the one who "feels" them and is the one best qualified to know whether they are relieved. When teaching is the nursing action to be evaluated, there must be evidence that the patient or family has learned what the nurse attempted to teach. The patient or family is the main source of data for evaluation of teaching—no one else can give the evidence that learning has taken place.

The physician helps evaluate the effectiveness of those nursing actions which he has prescribed, the dependent nursing functions delegated by him. In a collaborative team relationship the physician will also be concerned with evaluating independent nursing actions in terms of their contribution to the total care of the patient. Many nursing and medical functions are interdependent and work toward common goals so a mutual concern for evaluation is imperative. Likewise, other members of the health team (the physical therapist, dietitian, social service worker, others) collaborate in evaluating nursing actions which contribute to common goals for the patient. For instance, objectives relating to the patient's exercise or mobility might be shared by both nursing and physical therapy. The physical therapist may help evaluate the effectiveness of the nursing actions pertaining to exercise and mobility. It might be interjected here that physical therapists use several devices for measuring patient's exercise capacity which could be adapted for measuring the effectiveness of nursing care.

Evaluation Criteria

Use of measurable criteria for evaluating nursing care can contribute much toward the development of a science of nursing. These criteria will help in determining the predictability of results of nursing actions. To be of value to the developing profession, information regarding evaluation of nursing care must be shared. Sharing could be accomplished by systematically recording each step of the nursing process and the outcomes under varying conditions. The evolution of a science of nursing will be aided by a careful analysis and replication of the process by other nurses to lend validity and reliability to the findings.

Evaluation is based on objectives; it is the process by which one determines whether objectives have been reached. If the objectives are stated in such a way as to include the criteria by which achievement of the objective is determined, the evaluation is relatively simple. These criteria should indicate what the patient will be doing to show that the goal has been accomplished. The criteria will indicate the change in behavior which is expected as a result of nursing intervention.[1] Ideally these criteria should be measurable and should be recognized by a number of persons. In other words, if several nurses were to evaluate a nursing action, most of them would agree on their evaluation. The more objective and measurable the criteria for evaluation, the more reliable will be the results. Once

---

[1]See Chapter 5, section on Formulating Objectives, pp. 84-91.

these criteria have been established, evaluation consists of finding out if there is evidence that the desired change in behavior has occurred, if the patient is able to do what was hoped. There is room for partial achievement also.

While it is true that the present state of nursing is such that reliable criterion measures are either not known or not well developed, it is also likely that more are available to us than is realized. Perhaps some of the lack is because the profession has not come to grips with the need. It takes disciplined thinking to establish criteria for evaluating nursing care. It is quite possible that the development and confirmation of criterion measures is a contribution that nursing education can make to improve the practice of nursing. Teachers and students, who may have more time to devote to this process than practitioners, could establish criteria for common nursing objectives to serve as guides for the practitioner who can adapt the measures to the individual patient.

The more that is known about physiology and the psychosomatic interrelationships, the more use can be made of physiologic measures to evaluate various kinds of nursing care. Pulse rate and rhythm, respiratory rate, blood pressure, urine output, presence or absence of certain signs and symptoms, measure more than the obvious. As mentioned in Chapter 5, results of laboratory and X-ray examinations may serve as measures of nursing care. There is a great need for objective measures of emotional and social behavior, but progress can be made in this direction if the nurse will use descriptive, unambiguous terms to report behavior changes, and if she uses physiologic measures when appropriate. However, there are available some easy-to-use, short rating scales for evaluating various emotional states.[2] For some of these the interpretation of test results is explained well enough for nurses to use the tests in clinical situations. These rating scales and other psychometric tests might be useful in evaluating nursing care. For instance, the measure of depression could be administered to a depressed patient on admission and after a certain number of days of nursing care to see whether the nursing care produced measurable changes in the depression. Other therapies which might affect the depression should be controlled.

Types of criterion measures used should correspond to the desired outcomes of the nursing care. For instance, if a nursing objective is to reduce the work of the heart after a myocardial infarction, the nurse must consider the factors which comprise heart work. Two measures she might use are pulse rate and blood pressure. She would obtain these measures before and after a nursing action. If a ten percent variation were set as an acceptable limit, then the criteria by which she evaluates the actions are that the

[2]W. W. K. Zung, "A Self-Rating Depression Scale," *Archives of General Psychiatry*, 12:1(1965):63-70.

pulse rate varies less than ten percent from the resting rate, and the blood pressure (systolic, diastolic and/or pulse pressure) varies less than ten percent from the resting reading. When the nursing objective is related to teaching or counseling the patient, the nurse must ask herself what the patient will be doing and what change in his behavior will occur as a result of her teaching or counseling. To evaluate her teaching, the nurse asks the patient to perform the skill she has taught him while she observes his performance to see whether it is satisfactory. If the nurse teaches the patient a concept or counsels him regarding some aspect of health, she may ask the patient to reflect back what he has learned, or the nurse may observe the patient's behavior for evidence of desired changes. These actions or behaviors of the patient are criteria for evaluating teaching or counseling. As indicated earlier, these criteria are best selected when the objectives are formulated.

Outcomes of Evaluation

Whenever a nursing action is evaluated, the nurse must decide what to do about the findings of her evaluation. If a desired result is achieved, the actions should become part of the nursing care plan, especially if continuity of care is expected. Some nursing actions are for immediate goals and may only be needed for the moment. In this event, they need not be included in the written plan of care but should be added to the patient's record for future reference.

In the course of giving patient care, nursing actions may initiate a need for reassessment and another cycle of the nursing process. For instance, if the nurse gives a medication for the relief of pain, she will evaluate the effectiveness of this measure by whether the patient's pain is relieved. In addition, the nurse should consider the fact that analgesics have several effects on the patient, not only the desired effect but side effects and toxic reactions. The nurse must assess the patient for indications of the undesired effects as well as evaluate him for the desired effects. If some undesirable effects are present, additional nursing actions will need to be implemented and evaluated.

Once an objective is achieved and the problem no longer exists, the nursing actions prescribed for that objective should be deleted from the nursing care plan. If evaluation shows that the nursing actions did not achieve the goal or were too costly in terms of time, personnel, or materials, the nurse may need to look at alternative approaches to the goal and select another approach. The nursing care plan should reflect the change in approaches to the objective. The patient's record should indicate the change as well as the reason for the change.

Approaches to some objectives change with the physical or emotional status of the patient. Evaluation should indicate a need to change not only the approaches but the criteria by which they are measured. This is especially true of long-term goals. As the patient progresses, the overall objective may not change; the approaches may change, and the evaluation criteria may or may not change. For instance, refer again to the objective of reducing the work of the heart after a myocardial infarction. The criteria of ten percent change in heart rate and blood pressure may be used to evaluate the early attempts of the patient to feed himself or shave himself. The same criteria may be used later when he becomes ambulatory. When the patient goes home, his activity will be increased. Yet the same criteria may be used to determine how well he tolerates increased activity. As healing progresses, perhaps a twenty percent change in pulse rate and blood pressure would be acceptable limits. The objective of reducing the work of the heart has not changed. The actions changed as did the criteria.

McGuire[3] designed a tool for evaluating the nursing care of acutely and subacutely ill patients. It is not based on specific, personalized nursing objectives. It is an effective tool for evaluating personal hygiene and other general care of hospitalized patients. The nursing audit is a frequently used method of evaluating nursing care of discharged patients.[4] While this is a useful administrative device, it is not a substitute for the ongoing evaluation of nursing care. Evaluation of nursing care must be a continuous exercise if it is to aid in keeping the care suitable to the patient's needs.

Evaluation of nursing care is the step of the nursing process which determines the validity of nursing care—did it accomplish what it was designed to accomplish? It is as essential to the nursing process as any other step.

EVALUATION OF THE NURSING CARE PLAN

The chief purpose of a nursing care plan is to provide in written form a guide to the nursing care of the patient. This written plan must reflect all aspects of the patient's care and be written in such a way that all who use it will be able to follow it. The written plan must be up to date and must account for the changing needs of the patient as he progresses or as his condition worsens.

Each agency should establish criteria by which nursing care plans are evaluated. Using these criteria, the nursing care plans can be evaluated by the nurses who wrote them in order to improve their ability to write adequate plans. Administrative personnel may wish to evaluate nursing care plans from time to time to appraise the nurse's performance, to point out a

---

[3]Rita L. McGuire, "Bedside Nursing Audit," *American Journal of Nursing* 68:10 (1968):2146-2148.

[4]Maria C. Phaneuf, "A Nursing Audit Method," *Nursing Outlook* 12:5(1964): 42-45.

need for inservice education, or to judge the quality of nursing care being provided by the agency.

Some criteria for evaluating nursing care plans are presented in the accompanying guide. Details of each criterion could be developed for the agency in which it is used.

CRITERIA FOR EVALUATING NURSING CARE PLANS

1. Are the problems or needs a logical outcome of assessment data?
2. Are high priority problems indicated?
3. Are the goals appropriate to the problems identified?
4. Are both short- and long-term objectives stated? Are evaluation criteria included with the objectives?
5. Is there evidence that physical, mental, emotional, spiritual, social, and environmental needs were considered?
6. Do objectives pertain to prevention, therapy or palliation, and rehabilitation?
7. Do the nursing orders indicate:
   What is to be done?
   When it is to be done — specific hours?
   How it is adapted to the patient?
   Who is to do it?
8. Do the nursing actions represent a variety of nursing measures: comforting, teaching, counseling, referring, observing?
9. Is there a clear delineation of the responsibilities of the various members of the nursing team?
10. Are nursing responsibilities concerning the patient's appointments indicated?
11. Are the nursing measures related to medications and treatments specified as to methods of administration, effects to observe and report?
12. Does the plan reflect information from the nursing history and clinical inspection for personalizing care?
13. Does the plan indicate the patient's dependency level and how nursing promotes independence? Is the care consistent with patient's dependency level?
14. Is the nursing care plan up to date?
15. Is there a discharge plan?

REFERENCES

*ABDELLAH, FAYE. "Criterion Measures in Nursing." *Nursing Research* 10:1 (1961):21-6.

*CARN, IRENE. "The Nursing Audit as a Learning Tool for Undergraduates." *Nursing Clinics of North America* 4:2(1969):351-8.

Cash Area Conference. "*The Nursing Care Plan: A Basic Tool in Nursing Management.*" Los Angeles: Commission for Administrative Services in Hospitals. February, 1967.

*DAVID, HENRY P. "Some Criteria of Clinical Change and Measurement." *Journal of Psychiatric Nursing* 5:6(1967):550-4.

*McGUIRE, RETA L. "Bedside Nursing Audit." *American Journal of Nursing* 68:10(1968):2146-8.

NADLER, GERALD, and SAHNEY, VINOD. "A Descriptive Model of Nursing Case." *American Journal of Nursing* 69:2(1969):336-41.

NITE, GLADYS, and WILLIS, FRANK. *The Coronary Patient.* New York: The Macmillan Co., 1964.

*Suggested for additional reading.

*PHANEUF, MARK C. "Analysis of a Nursing Audit." *Nursing Outlook* 16:1 (1968):57-60.

*—— "The Nursing Audit for Evaluation of Patient Care." *Nursing Outlook* 14:6(1966):51-4.

*—— "A Nursing Audit Method." *Nursing Outlook* 12:5(1964):42-5.

CLINICAL EXPERIENCE

1. Critically evaluate the objectivity of the criterion measures used to evaluate the nursing care of one or more patients.
2. Try out some criterion measures used for objectives concerned with emotional, spiritual, or social needs by having two or three nurses evaluate the care. Check the results of the evaluations for agreement.
3. Using the Criteria for Evaluation of a Nursing Care Plan, evaluate two or three nursing care plans. Write out a constructive criticism of one nursing care plan.
4. Follow through on the results of evaluation of several nursing actions which were ineffective. Under what circumstances was an alternative approach used without reassessing the patient? Under what circumstances was a reappraisal of the patient's problem necessary?

*Suggested for additional reading.

Chapter 8

Theory Into Practice

At several points in the preceding chapters, mention has been made of the scientific principles basic to nursing and of the importance of planning patient care based on scientific principles. The presentation of the nursing process in the planning of patient care would not be complete without a discussion of the theoretical basis of nursing practice.

Nursing is a person-to-person encounter between the nurse and an individual who needs her services. Nursing care is derived from a wide variety of sources made available to the nurse by education and experience. The unique caring component of nursing originates in the nurse's appreciation of the individuality of the person and the meanings that life and health have for him. Her appreciation of the other person is derived from the nurse's own philosophy of life, her beliefs about the nature of man and the meanings of life. Her value systems stem from her cultural and religious background and her education. A study of the humanities helps the nurse gain insight into the nature of man, his value, and his contribution to society. If nursing care is patient-centered, the nurse must be willing to know and to respect the uniqueness of the individual patient and to plan his care with this uniqueness in mind. To plan patient care, the nurse must draw on all the resources at her command if the care is representative of both the art and the science of nursing.

THEORETICAL BASIS OF NURSING

Many nursing educators believe that there is theory unique to nursing but that little has been accomplished toward identification of nursing theory. Nursing also borrows concepts, theories, and principles from other sciences and applies them in ways different from other health professions. In a sense, the unique ways in which nursing applies these concepts is the science of nursing.

In general, nursing theory can be developed in two ways. One method is to analyze carefully collected clinical data to ascertain relationships between cause and effect or between changes in patient behavior and nursing care. From this analysis, hypotheses are formulated and tested in clinical practice. The outcomes of hypothesis testing in relation to different variables can lead to the development of nursing theory. This method would be more likely to establish nursing as an independent discipline than would other methods.[1] One reason for nurses to be objective, comprehensive, and precise in observing and recording patient behavior and the results of nursing actions is to furnish data for analysis which could lead to unique nursing theory.

The other method of developing nursing theory is to examine concepts and principles from other sciences in order to determine their usefulness for nursing. This method could be wasteful of time and energy as nurses search through the concepts and principles of other disciplines to find some which have relevance for nursing. Fortunately, a number of nurses have pursued graduate study in various disciplines and they can serve the profession by identifying relevant concepts from their particular field of interest.

A method of applying concepts from behavioral and natural sciences to nursing is described below for those nurses who have not yet developed their own methods of applying theory to practice. Since both under-graduate and graduate nurses study courses which are applicable to nursing, they should know how to discover and apply various concepts to nursing.

Regardless of the sources of nursing knowledge, the nurse must first have a clear picture of what nursing is, what the independent functions of nursing are. She needs to combine her ideas about nursing with a fair amount of creativity and imagination so that nursing measures might be originated as an application of the principle or concept. There are a number of questions the nurse might ask as she endeavors to discover nursing measures which apply various principles and concepts.

Is there a relationship between this principle or concept and

- the various aspects of personal hygiene?
- the posture and position of the patient?
- the timing and organization of patient care?
- the patient's environment: temperature, humidity, sanitation, microbiology?
- social, cultural, and religious influences on the person's behavior?
- the social milieu in which the patient is?
- nutrition: the food and fluids available in kind, amount, consistency, frequency of intake?
- the exercise or activity level of the patient?
- the health practices of the person or family?

---

[1]Florence S. Wald and Robert C. Leonard, "Towards Development of Nursing Practice Theory, *Nursing Research* 13:4(1964):309-313.

Does this principle or concept suggest

- observations of significance to the patient's progress?
- ways to decrease stress or anxiety, conflict, frustration?
- need to stimulate or depress a body function?
- methods of providing comfort, rest, relaxation?
- ways to improve communication?
- ways of preventing complications of disease?
- ways of promoting positive health?
- methods for understanding and helping people cope with their reactions to illness, hospitalization, therapy, rehabilitation?
- ways of preventing disease or exacerbations of a disease?
- methods for studying human behavior which could be used for nursing research or for evaluation of nursing care?

Looking for answers to these questions while studying in any field of knowledge can give the nurse new ideas to test in nursing practice.

Application of Behavioral Science

Knowledge of psychology, sociology, and anthropology that the nurse has may help her understand behavior and group relationships and the constraints placed upon people by the groups to which they belong. Behavioral sciences help the nurse realize that people cope with stress and anxiety in unique ways which have meaning to the individual.

If nurses are to be change agents, they must understand how change is effected and how people react to change. Behavioral sciences explain the fact that people find change difficult. For change to take place, the change must be acceptable to the person. The nurse must also accept the fact that change usually occurs over a period of time rather than momentarily. People cling to their customary patterns of behaving, and these must be considered and appreciated if nursing care involves change.

A knowledge of normal growth and development of the human being through his total life span gives the nurse an indication of how well the patient has developed in relation to norms. It also helps her understand some of the problems peculiar to certain age groups, the risks to health faced at any one stage of development. The nurse, operating from a broad basis of knowledge, is often able to plan care to forestall development of many health/illness problems.

Some behavioral science concepts which have relevance for nursing include role development, role change, culture as a determinant of behavior, coping behavior, authority and power, group behavior, stress, space, privacy.

Application of psychosocial concepts to nursing follows a pattern of thinking from cause to effect to utilization. When a nurse thinks that a certain concept has relevance for nursing, she might ask herself (or the teacher might ask the student) several questions. To illustrate the application of a behavorial science concept to nursing, the concept of body image will be briefly described in terms of these questions.

"Under what circumstances does the concept apply to human behavior?"

Body image is the mental picture that a person has of his body. It is an aspect of human personality, normally outside conscious awareness. Disturbances in body image occur when the person fails to see and adapt to his body and its parts as they actually are. Disturbances in body image are precipitated by loss or disease of a body part, disfigurement, loss of a body function, defect or deformity of a body part, degenerative changes.[2]

"If these circumstances are present for a particular patient, what data support their existence?"

Identify data regarding any of the precipitating causes of disturbances of body image. Look for data concerning the person's attitudes regarding his body and his adaptations to changes in his body.

"According to the concept, how do people behave when the concept is operational?"

Acceptance of changed body image is shown by willingness to discuss the disturbance, and ability to accept help.

Responses to body image disturbances include anxiety, grief and mourning, denial, prolonged depression, hostility, failure to accept help and work toward rehabilitation.

"Does the patient behave in a typical way?"

Assess the patient's behavior for clues about his attitudes, feelings, thoughts regarding the changes in his body.

"If desirable adaptive behavior may occur when the concept is operational, what can be done to facilitate the adaptive behavior? What do other disciplines do to help people adapt, and which methods are suitable for nurses to use?"

Engle,[3] Thaler,[4] and Ujheley[5] describe ways that nurses can help people in the various stages of mourning, which is "normal" behavior when a disturbance of body image occurs. Some ways of dealing with various phases of mourning include:

Denial—accept, but do not reinforce.

Sadness—do not be gay and lighthearted; this can accentuate the person's sadness. Care for him in such a way as to show he is a person of worth, his body is still worth taking care of. Good grooming fosters this feeling. Be concerned about what the person is concerned about.

---

[2]Lawrence Kolb, "Disturbances of the Body-Image," *American Handbook of Psychiatry,* Vol. 1, Silvano Arieti, ed. (New York: Basic Books, 1959), pages 749-769.

[3]George L. Engle, "Grief and Grieving," *American Journal of Nursing* 64:9(1964): 93-98.

[4]Otto F. Thaler, "Grief and Depression," Nursing Forum II(1966):9-22.

[5]Gertrude Ujheley, "Grief and Depression: Implications for Preventive and Therapeutic Nursing Care," *Nursing Forum* II(1966):23-25.

Facing reality—explore with the patient the meaning of his loss, the implications in terms of his life patterns. Sensory stimulation techniques may be beneficial with some kinds of loss (amputations, paralysis). Use touch to reinforce the reality of the loss.

"If undesirable behavior may occur when this concept is operational, what can be done to prevent or attenuate the maladaptive behavior? What do other disciplines do to help people substitute adaptive for maladaptive behavior? Which methods are suitable for nurses to use?"

Pathophysiological responses to altered body image include prolonged denial and depression, failure to reorganize the body image, and inability to follow a rehabilitation program. Counseling approaches and referrals are used when these responses occur. Nurses can support the counselor's approaches.

"In what ways do other disciplines evaluate change in behavior when the concept is operational? Which of these ways are suitable or adaptable for evaluation of nursing care?"

Rorschach tests, Draw-a-Person tests, Secord's Homonym test, self-rating depression scales, and others, as well as objective observations of behavior are used to study disturbances of body image. All but the first of these might be used by nurses.

Since nursing is a person-to-person encounter, the more the nurse knows about behavioral sciences, the more she will understand and be able to help the people she serves.

Application of Natural Science

Among the natural sciences which have relevance for nursing are physiology, anatomy, chemistry, physics, nutrition, pathology, and epidemiology. In order for the nurse to identify health/illness problems, she should understand what health is and what impairments of health may occur. The nurse's knowledge of physiology, anatomy, and nutrition gives her a basis for estimating physical health as well as determining needs for the maintenance of health.

Chemistry and physics are essential to an understanding of physiology and nutrition as well as pharmacology. Many of the principles upon which nursing actions are based derive from chemistry, physics, and microbiology.

The medical sciences acquaint the nurse with the causes and effects of disease and the usual therapy. Her knowledge of medical and other sciences gives the nurse a basis for initiating preventive measures, for recognizing and interpreting signs and symptoms of disease, for proposing alternative measures to relieve discomforts, and for evaluating the patient's progress.

Physiology.

Nursing care to relieve a symptom or change a patho-physiological manifestation is based on an understanding of physiology. In order to utilize physiology in nursing practice, the nurse must consider the various factors controlling the function in question.

An example concerning the problem of nausea might serve to illustrate the application of physiology to nursing practice. Nausea is due to the stimulation of the vomiting center by way of sensory nerves or the chemoreceptor trigger zone. [6, 7] Sensory nerves relaying information to the vomiting (nausea) center are diffuse and multiple.

"What evidence indicates that the function is not operating normally?"

Nausea and vomiting are protective mechanisms designed to rid the body of noxious substances. Nausea only occurs as a result of noxious stimuli. Identify a disease process, a circulating chemical, or other stimulus to the vomiting center.

"What is the evidence of malfunction in the patient?"

Possible clues might be: discomfort, inability to take food or fluid, pallor, sweating, salivation. The verbal complaint of nausea is indisputable evidence.

"What are the possible ways the function can be stimulated?"

Postnasal pressure; distention of the stomach, small intestine, or biliary tract; distention or injury to uterus, renal pelvis, or bladder; increased intracranial pressure; stimulation of semicircular canals (motion sickness); many kinds of pain, unpleasant sights, smells, tastes, or sensations; exogenous or endogenous toxins; irritating substances in the gastrointestinal tract; circulating drugs; emotional disturbances.

"What are the possible ways the function can be depressed?"

Anti-emetic drugs raise the threshold for afferent impulses to the center.

"What factors controlling the function are operating in the patient?"

To find out which of the above are operating in a particular patient, the nurse can seek answers to these questions:

—Has the patient had an anesthetic or drug which produces nausea as a side effect?
—Is the nausea related to the time of administration of some drug or treatment?
—Is the patient receiving drugs which leave a bad taste in his mouth?
—Are there any disagreeable sights, smells, tastes, sensations being experienced by the patient?
—Is the patient emotionally upset? What happened to him just before he became nauseated?
—Does the patient have pain?
—Does the patient have a tumor, swelling, or fluid pressing on internal organs or distending them?
—Does his disease process produce toxins?

"Which factors controlling the function can be removed, attenuated, or facilitated by nursing actions?"

6Arthur C. Guyton, *Textbook of Medical Physiology* (Philadelphia: W. B. Saunders Co., 1966), pp. 924-926.

7T. R. Harrison, *et al.* (eds.), *Principles of Internal Medicine*, (New York: McGraw-Hill Book Company, 1966), pp. 108-110.

Some nursing actions which might result from the answers to the above questions follow:

—Induce vomiting to remove irritating substances from stomach.
—If drug-related, discuss effect with physician.
—Remove soiled, odorous dressings, flowers, drainage, emesis basins, bedpans.
—Deodorize the room.
—Give opportunity to talk out emotional problems, possibly give a sedative or some nursing measure to relax the patient, such as a back rub.
—Measures to relieve pain, special attention that analgesic is not the cause of nausea.
—Positioning to relieve pressure of tumors or distended organs.
—Check functioning of nasogastric suction.
—Anti-emetic drugs to raise threshold of the center; (not an indedendent nursing measure).
—Teaching about cause and effect relationships, prevention, ways to diminish sensation of nausea and prevent vomiting.

"What are the possible effects if the malfunction continues? What measures can nurses use to prevent or attenuate these effects?"

Fluid and electrolyte imbalances, malnutrition. Nurses can obtain prescription for parenteral fluids, dietary supplements. Teach patient about adequate nutrition when symptom subsides.

"What methods are used to study this function? Which ones might nurses use to evaluate nursing care?"

The multiplicity of variables causing nausea makes it a difficult symptom to study clinically. However, careful recording of the data about the patient, showing which variables are operating in that patient, and observation of the effects of nursing measures could lead to more specific knowledge regarding the specificity of various nursing measures in the relief of the symptom. Noting the effect of the symptom on the vital signs and the changes in vital signs when various relief measures are used could be used to study the effects of nausea.

Study of physiology can awaken the nurse to new and interesting ways of relieving the signs and symptoms of disease as well as promoting health. Such a study might shatter some traditional nursing concepts, but it could also invest the simple acts of nursing with considerable therapeutic value.

Physics, Chemistry, Microbiology.

The laws and principles of physics, chemistry, and microbiology should be examined in terms of the component variables. Nursing measures can manipulate some of the variables in order to achieve desired ends. A few examples of the application of principles of these sciences will suffice to illustrate their value for nursing.

For instance, consider the physical principle regarding the dosage of radioactivity which varies directly with time of exposure and inversely with the square of the distance between source and object.[8] When planning the care of a patient being treated with a radioactive substance, nurses can protect themselves from radioactivity by decreasing the time they are with the patient and by increasing the distance between them and the patient.

Many other physical laws and principles have relevance for nursing. The variables effecting the behavior of gases, the volume, temperature, and pressure, are manipulated by a number of nursing actions. These laws are particularly applicable to the care of patients with respiratory problems.

Chemical reactions are known to occur more rapidly as the temperature of the reactants is increased.[9] This principle helps nurses understand the effects on body metabolism during fever or hypothermia. This principle is also utilized in hastening or slowing the action of a medication by altering the temperature of the diluent.

It is known that microorganisms multiply only when food, oxygen, moisture, and other conditions are present.[10] In controlling the spread of communicable disease, in aseptic techniques, and in other methods of protecting people from infectious organisms, nurses remove or alter one or more of the conditions essential for the growth of microorganisms.

A knowledge of natural sciences not only supplies explanations for what the nurse does but it also can give her a basis for designing new and better methods of manipulating the environment to improve patient care. Knowledge of these sciences, too, might lead to questioning some traditional nursing practices and to pointing out a need to base nursing practice on science rather than tradition.

A CHALLENGE

Challenges of nursing are many. One challenge arises from the application of scientific principles through each step of the nursing process, thereby strengthening the foundations of nursing. Another challenge is presented by being able to predict outcomes of nursing care so well that behaviorally stated objectives have a high probability of success. To help persons maintain their integrity in times of crisis is another exciting undertaking for nurses. Not all patients recover, yet nurses may have the high privilege of being with people in the last stages of life and helping them to find meaning and wholeness even in this experience. Perhaps the greatest challenge lies in motivating people to live healthfully so as to prevent disease and assure a more abundant life.

---

[8]Maud E. Greenwood, *Medical Physics* (Philadelphia: F. A. Davis Co., 1963), p. 28.

[9]Linus Pauling, *College Chemistry* (San Francisco: W. H. Freeman, 1956), pp. 406-407.

[10]Alice Lorraine Smith, *Microbiology and Pathology* (St. Louis: C. V. Mosby Co., 1964), p. 61.

Planning of patient care which is personalized to the individual patient offers a challenge to the professional nurse. The planning of patient care is a dynamic, stimulating experience. It brings the nurse in contact with unique individuals and families who need the help that she can give. A careful assessment of the person's needs leads to a personalized plan of care which helps the patient cope with his health/illness problems in such a way as to promote his optimal well-being. Much of the satisfaction the nurse derives from her work will be due to the successful outcomes of the plans she has fashioned. Thoughtful, intelligent planning based on a meaningful relationship with patients and/or families should produce measurable changes in their health/illness status. Seeing these changes and helping people toward a more abundant life can provide the nurse with the incentive she needs to grow in professional competence, to become more skillful in planning patient care.

Assessment, intervention, evaluation. These constitute the process of nursing. Expertness in the use of the nursing process improves with knowledge and experience. When the nursing process is used in planning patient care, nursing can contribute to the health care of people in such a way as to meet the person's needs and to promote their health. In addition, the practice of nursing must advance the development of the nurse herself as well as the profession to which she belongs. Both the humanitarian and the scientific aspects of nursing will be advanced by the systematic use of the nursing process in the planning of patient care.

REFERENCES

BECK, A. T. *et al.* "An Inventory for Measuring Depression." *Archives of General Psychiatry* 4:6(1961):561-71.

BENNIS, W. G. *et al.* *The Planning of Change.* New York: Holt, Rinehart and Winston, Inc. 1969.

*BROWN, ESTHER L. *Newer Dimensions of Patient Care.* New York: Russell Sage Foundation. 1965.

BROWN, MYRTLE IRENE. "Social Theory in Geriatric Nursing Research." *Nursing Research* 17:3(1968):213-7.

CLELAND, VIRGINIA S. "The Use of Existing Theories." *Nursing Research* 16:2(1967):118:21.

CONANT, LUCY M. "Closing the Practice-Theory Gap." *Nursing Outlook* 15:11 (1967):37-9.

*CROCKER, GOLDIE. "Nursing in a Sociological Perspective." *Nursing Outlook* 16:4(1968):65-7.

*ELLIS, ROSEMARY. "Characteristics of Significant Theories." *Nursing Research* 17:3(1968):217-22.

*ENGLE, GEORGE L. "Grief and Grieving." *American Journal of Nursing* 64:9 (1964):93-8.

*FOLTA, JEANETTE R. "Perspectives of an Applied Scientist." *Nursing Research* 17:6(1968)502-5.

*Suggested for additional reading.

GREENWOOD, MAUD E. *Medical Physics*. Philadelphia: F. A. Davis Co. 1963.
GUYTON, ARTHUR C. *Textbook of Medical Physiology*. Philadelphia: W. B. Saunders Co. 1966.
HARRISON, T. R. *et al.* (Eds.). *Principles of Internal Medicine*. New York: McGraw-Hill Book Company. 1966.
*JOHNSON, DOROTHY E. "Theory in Nursing: Borrowed and Unique." *Nursing Research* 17:3(1968):206-9.
KOLB, LAWRENCE C. "Disturbances of the Body-Image." *American Handbook of Psychiatry*. Vol. I. Silvano Arieti, ed. New York: Basic Books, Inc. (1959): 749-69.
McCAIN, R. FAYE. "Systematic Investigation of Medical Surgical Nursing Content." *Journal of Nursing Education* 4:2(1965):23-31.
*MOORE, MARJORIE A. "Nursing: A Scientific Discipline?" *Nursing Forum* VII:4 (1968):340-8.
*NORRIS, CATHERINE M. "Toward a Science of Nursing." *Nursing Forum* III:3: (1964):10-44.
OSBORNE, OLIVER H. "Anthropology and Nursing: Some Common Traditions and Interests." *Nursing Research* 18:3(1969):251-5.
QUINT, JEANNE C. "The Case for Theories Generated from Empirical Data." *Nursing Research* 16:2(1967):109-14.
*RUBIN, REVA. "A Theory of Clinical Nursing." *Nursing Research* 17:3(1968): 210-12.
*SCHRAG, CLARENCE. "Science and the Helping Professions." *Nursing Research* 17:6(1968):486-96.
SMITH, ALICE LORRAINE. *Microbiology and Pathology*, St. Louis: C. V. Mosby Co. 1964.
Systems and Procedures Association, "Operations Research," *Business Systems*. Cleveland: Systems and Procedures Association, Chap. 21, 22:(1966):1-33.
*THALER, OTTO F. "Grief and Depression." *Nursing Forum* V:2(1966):9-22.
*UJHELEY, GERTRUDE. "Grief and Depression: Implications for Preventive and Therapeutic Nursing Care." *Nursing Forum* V-2(1966):23-35.
*WALD, FLORENCE S., and LEONARD, ROBERT C. "Towards Development of Nursing Practice Theory." *Nursing Research*. 13(Fall, 1964):309-13.
*WATTS, WILMA. "Social Class, Ethnic Background and Patient Care." *Nursing Forum* VI:2(1967):155-62.
ZUNG, W. W. K. "A Self-Rating Depression Scale." *Archives of General Psychiatry* 12:1(1965):63-70.

CLINICAL EXPERIENCE

1. Conduct a clinical research project of your own selection.
2. Do library research on a concept or principle from a behavorial or natural science. Outline its application to nursing practice. Try it on a number of patients. Tabulate and analyze your findings. Draw conclusions. Submit a paper for publication.

*Suggested for additional reading.

INDEX